EXPERIENCING HIV

Experiencing HIV

PERSONAL, FAMILY, AND WORK RELATIONSHIPS

BARRY D. ADAM
AND
ALAN SEARS

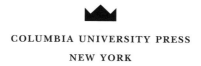

COLUMBIA UNIVERSITY PRESS

NEW YORK

Columbia University Press
Publishers Since 1893
New York   Chichester, West Sussex
Copyright © 1996 Columbia University Press
All rights reserved

Library of Congress Cataloging-in-Publication Data
Adam, Barry D.
    Experiencing HIV : personal, family, and work relationships /
    Barry D. Adam and Alan Sears
        p. cm.
    Includes bibliographical references and index.
    ISBN 0-231-10120-1 (cl : alk. paper). – ISBN 0-231-10121-X (pa :
alk. paper)
    1. HIV-positive persons–Interviews.   I. Sears. Alan.   II. Title.
RC607.A26A34185   1996
362.1'969792–dc20   96-19248
                                                           CIP

Casebound editions of Columbia University Press books are printed on permanent and
durable acid-free paper.

Printed in the United States of America

c 10 9 8 7 6 5 4 3 2 1
p 10 9 8 7 6 5 4 3 2 1

CONTENTS

PREFACE

The idea for this book came about in the course of our involvement with community-based AIDS work. Our concern about AIDS began with the first identification of the syndrome in 1981: along with other early activists, we never felt the luxury of considering ourselves unaffected by the epidemic. Before the invention of the HIV-antibody test, none of us knew who would be conscripted next into the syndrome as our friends and lovers developed symptoms one after the other. One of us was among the founders of the first organized response to AIDS in his community and both of us have served numerous roles in the education and support work of the local organization. As sociologists, we were struck by the paucity of research of direct use to frontline workers and to people living with AIDS. The first step we took in developing this project was to talk at length with several HIV-positive people about the issues which concern them most and about which they would be most interested in reading. We found a range of outstanding concerns that were not being met by the rapidly increasing flow of advice books, seminars, and professional workshops aimed at people in the syndrome.

We went to the experts to find the answers to these questions and so interviewed 100 seropositive people and their caregivers in southeastern

Michigan and southwestern Ontario who were black and white, male and female, gay and heterosexual, well off and poor, American and Canadian. A précis of the results appeared in a 41-page handbook entitled *People With HIV/AIDS Talk . . . About Life, Love, Work, and Family* which we distributed to HIV-positive people through the many organizations which assisted us in this project. In 1994, the Ontario Ministry of Health provided us with a grant to distribute the handbook through all of the community-based AIDS organizations in the province and the handbook remains available through the AIDS Committee of Windsor, P.O. Box 2233, Windsor, Ontario, Canada N8Y 4R8. While the handbook offers a taste of the many rich narratives of people experiencing HIV, this book offers the full menu.

This study could not have been realized without the invaluable assistance of John R. Dufour in organizing and transcribing interviews and through the support of Rev. Joseph Harmon and Vanessa Smith; the following AIDS service organizations: AIDS Committee of Windsor, Wellness Networks, Community Health Awareness Group, Friends Alliance, Wellness House, AIDS Care Connection, Children's Immune Disorder, and La Casa (now Latino) Family Services; and the financial support of the Canadian Foundation for AIDS Research and the University of Windsor Research Board. Barry Adam benefitted from a Research Professorship granted by the University of Windsor. We are also grateful for the advice and assistance of the people in support groups who commented on the handbook, and to the following people who read drafts of the book in progress: Glenn Schellenberg, Stephen Murray, Jacqueline Lewis, Kevin Mumford, Eleanor Maticka Tyndale, and John R. Dufour. We benefitted a good deal from having readers drawn from several disciplines who, like the study participants, are men and women, white and black, HIV-positive and negative, and gay, lesbian, and heterosexual. Portions of the Introduction and Chapter 4 have appeared in the journal, *Medical Anthropology* (Adam and Sears 1994) and early versions of other parts have been presented to the Canadian Sociology and Anthropology Association in Charlottetown and Montreal, the American Sociological Association in Washington, and the Queer Sites conference in Toronto.

The completion of this project was not always easy given the resistance of government institutions to funding research that takes seriously the lives of people with AIDS outside of a medical context and that crosses national boundaries. We were detained and interrogated by United States immigration officials on three occasions. On finding that we were visiting AIDS-related social service agencies or were speaking with HIV-positive people, they demanded to know whether we were HIV-positive in accord with the U.S. law forbidding the entry of HIV-positive people into the country.[1]

While we both contributed to the design, carrying out, and authorship of this project and book, we did have a division of labor in writing first drafts so that Barry Adam wrote Chapters 3, 4, 5, and the Conclusion, and Alan Sears wrote Chapters 1, 2, 6, and 7.

INTRODUCTION

These are stories about the effects of HIV infection on personal, family, and work relationships. Indeed the burdens associated with the social aspects of AIDS and HIV may outweigh physical problems for many people coping with immunodeficiency syndrome, especially those with few or no symptoms. In offering these narratives about living with HIV, we have two fundamental objectives. The first is to "give voice" to people with HIV infection in order to identify the everyday problems associated with the disease, to describe them, and to talk about working them through. Our intent in doing this is "to facilitate a culture of coping strategies, success stories, and practical knowledge for managing the disease" (Adam 1992b:13) and thus to help build knowledge of direct interest and use for seropositive people themselves. This book is intended not simply to create knowledge *about* people with HIV but to create knowledge *for* people with HIV. The second objective is to reflect upon these stories about living with HIV to see how the people most directly affected by the epidemic make sense of AIDS and structure lives through these narratives.

This book focuses on *living* with HIV disease and AIDS to show the many ways in which people deal, adequately or inadequately, with the difficulties posed by the syndrome. Our interest is less in the biographies of the particular people who participated in this study than in the coping strategies they employed. These chapters do not so much *look back* on the personalities of individuals to explain why they chose the coping strategies they did, but rather offer a menu of possibilities that readers might take up in *looking forward* to dealing with similar situations. Participants in this study provide a wealth of creative responses in addressing such problems as forming intimate relationships with new people, disclosing to family members, and holding a job. Their stories are much more than the responses of single individuals or of doctor-patient relationships which are the focus of so many studies reliant on clinical samples. Caregivers, friends, lovers, and household members must also live with HIV in their own ways and their experiences are documented here.

When physicians confront disease, they do not directly face a pathogen, but rather they gather together patients' reports about their experiences and "read" bodily symptoms as effects of an underlying cause. Sociologists are concerned with not only the potential physiological development of an illness but also the work involved in its management, the impact of illness, and the changes in the lives of the ill and their families that in turn affect their management of the illness itself (Corbin and Strauss 1988:47–48).

The approach of this book to "experiencing HIV" is, then, not a display of physical suffering, but one of showing how HIV affects social relationships and how social relationships, in turn, affect living with HIV. Just as HIV acts biologically to undermine protective immunological defenses against a range of once-benign, preexisting conditions, it may also act socially to expose unresolved tensions in personal relationships once managed by ad hoc adjustments and the norms of civility.

An HIV-positive diagnosis disturbs patterns of belief about oneself and the world, as well as physical and personal relations. Michael Bury (1982:169) uses the term "biographical disruption" to describe the impact of chronic illness "where the structures of everyday life and the forms of knowledge which underpin them are disrupted." This biographical disruption forces an examination of many of the taken-for-granted assumptions upon which lives are built, and leads to a reconstruction of one's own biography, as well as a reformulation of intentions, plans, and personal projects. Just how lives are pieced "back" together depends on the resources and choices that can be brought to the situation. Biographical reconstruction depends on material resources such as job security and access to medical services; it depends on social support provided by caregivers; and it is shaped by the ideas and stories available for making sense of what has happened and identifying solutions to HIV-related problems. All of these factors shape perceptions of the available options and influence the choices that must be made day to day. Even the decision to simply carry on as before is a way of living with HIV which must be reconstituted amid new meanings and negotiated around new constraints or uncertainties.

Making a life with HIV is an active process of developing ways of dealing with actual or anticipated changes in self or others in areas ranging from physical health to intimacy or employment. People with HIV have been "present at their own making": individually and collectively they have challenged medicine, the state, and the common sense of the day to work out ways of living with a condition that many in society still label a "death sentence"—with all of its punitive connotations. [1]

Peter Sedgwick (1982:32) argues, "there are no illnesses or diseases in nature," meaning that people or institutions must deem particular conditions to be either healthy and normal, or unhealthy and deviant. A condition considered to be a sign of ill-health in one setting (e.g. seeing visions) might be seen in entirely different terms (e.g. as the mark of a prophet) in another. Illness is not, however, *simply* a social construction. People face very real pain, impairment, and destruction in coping with disease, but it is only through specific social processes that these effects become identified as the product of illness as opposed to, for example, the outcome of aging, the wages of sin, or the mark of exceptionalness. The memory loss of an elderly person, for example, might be considered to be a natural part of the aging process or the particular devastation wrought by a specific disease.[2] We learn something, then, by understanding the social circumstances under which a particular set of changes is identified with a specific illness.

Capitalist societies tend to define health in terms of the capacity to perform certain tasks, particularly the work expected as a result of one's position in society. Illness, as a result, is something which impairs work performance, whether in the form of paid employment, unpaid work in the household, or related undertakings such as education. This "functional" definition contrasts with an "experiential" definition where people feel themselves to be ill to the extent to which they cannot control their bodies and their lives to meet their self-defined needs and desires (Doyal 1979:34–35; Berliner 1977:117). According to the functional definition (Parsons 1951), illness is problematic, as it prevents people from performing their social roles. Illness functions as a temporary role position to control this threat to the social system by exempting individ-

uals from regular duties on the condition that they are genuinely ill and
are doing their utmost to get well. The sick role is thus a means of regulation which protects the integrity of the system of role obligations by
allowing a temporary release only under specified conditions. The social
requirement to fulfill role expectations is reinforced by specifying the
particular conditions for temporary respite.

It flows from the functional definition that objective measures must
exist for genuine illness. Impairment must be certified from the outside
in order to qualify as a legitimate pretext for exemption from duties.
This certification, in Parsons' (1951:437) words, "has the social function
of protection against 'malingering.' " Scientific medicine is charged with
providing these "objective" measures. Indeed, these external criteria are
privileged over the experience that ill people have of their own bodies
and minds. Michael Taussig (1992:99) argues, "the clinical situation
becomes a combat zone of disputes over power and over definitions of
illness and degrees of incapacity."

One of the characteristics of illness across cultures is a "quest for
explanation" (Sedgwick 1982:35). The changes ill people experience
are explained in various terms, ranging from contemporary germ theory to accounts of spiritual possession. Scientific medicine is unique
among the explanatory systems humans have developed for illness in its
insistence on the objective character of both the disease process and our
knowledge of it. The specific social content of scientific medicine is
denied, so that categories that arise out of specific social relations
(healthy or normal, genuine illness, tolerable or intolerable pain) are
presented as facts of nature (Taussig 1992; Tesh 1988).

Illness, in the functional definition of illness, is at once considered
instrumentally, as the impairment of task performance, and *morally*, as
deviation from norms of conduct, whether legitimate or not.[3] It is thus
not a unique feature of living with HIV that illness is inflected with a
moral content. Any illness in contemporary capitalist society may be
seen as suspect insofar as it exempts people from the everyday grind of
paid employment or household labor. Further, illness is integrally connected to marginality in that the individuals who cannot perform
expected tasks will tend to lose both the material benefits of work and
the sense of self that may be connected with doing their jobs in the workforce or the home.[4] The moral element of blaming the victim in cases of
illness flows from a set of social relations in which individuals are seen as
responsible for maintaining their own bodies and minds at levels of fit-
ness required *externally* (e.g. by employers). The moral attributions of
blame associated with AIDS have been particularly intense given the links

to groups facing specific forms of discrimination and marginalization. People making a life with HIV must therefore negotiate both the general moral dimensions of illness and the specific attributions associated with AIDS. They must also contend with an externally imposed functional definition of illness that may or may not line up with their own self-defined experiential measures of well-being.

A rich research literature has developed examining the social construction of AIDS since its "discovery" in 1981. This body of work illuminates the social processes through which AIDS has been used to exploit inequalities based on sexual orientation, race, class, and gender (Patton 1985; Altman 1986; Watney 1987; Crimp 1988; Clatts and Mutchler 1989; Carter and Watney 1989; Adam 1992a; Patton 1994). It has been widely noted that scant attention has been paid to issues of living with HIV for seropositive people and their friends and families (Tiblier 1987:259; Cleveland et al. 1988:154; Lovejoy 1990:311; Siegel and Krauss 1991:18; Pierret 1992:67–68). Work on the subjectivity of AIDS is comparatively preliminary (see Weitz 1991; Shelby 1992; O'Brien 1992; Brown and Powell-Cope 1992).[5] This book delineates the ways in which people with HIV themselves make lives for themselves in the context of specific social relations and cultural constructions of AIDS.

Constructing AIDS

Coping with HIV disease has never been simply an issue of dealing with the physical consequences of illness. The ways in which AIDS has been taken up as a public issue have helped shape the attitudes of families and co-workers, the expectations of household members, and certainly the initial apprehensions of seropositive people themselves. After AIDS was first identified in North America in 1981, it quickly became part of a highly charged sociopolitical milieu which shaped its trajectory and meanings over the ensuing years. At first consigned to the oblivion imposed upon all things associated with gay, black, and poor people, it later fell prey to an inundation of speculation, terror, and moral entrepreneurship in the mid-1980s. AIDS raised fundamental human anxieties about sex and death, and entered history in the midst of "a period of conflict over the (dis)establishment of the nuclear family and the rights of people to take up new domestic and sexual arrangements outside the purview of patriarchal authority" (Adam 1992a:305).

As AIDS was first identified in North America among gay men, drug users, African Americans, and Latinos—all groups traditionally underrepresented in or excluded from the political system—much of the subsequent debate over control of HIV transmission became a conflict over who gets to control whose bodies. Conservatives tended to view safer sex, like abortion and contraception before it, as "yet another sign of the decline of the nuclear family because it allowed the escape of sex from family control, it released women from the obligations of motherhood and into the labor market, it permitted men to have sex while avoiding the responsibilities of family, and it let sex 'leak away' from the family to youth and to people who might stay unmarried, become 'loose' or 'bad' women, or prefer homosexual relationships" (Adam 1992a:308–309). Moral entrepreneurs rapidly took AIDS as a symbolic weapon in the restoration of "traditional values," "the" family, and monogamy. Public discourse constructed white, middle class, heterosexuals as the innocent self threatened by a guilty other of "AIDS carriers." Governments typically responded to AIDS in the early 1980s with a refusal to act, delay, or neglect, or very tentative initiatives aimed less at assisting those afflicted with AIDS than protecting an ostensibly unafflicted "general public" (Adam 1992a).

The voices of people with the disease were very often submerged by a tide of competing forces which sought to give AIDS a meaning to their own liking. The limited public avenues permitted by the mass media for the expression of experiences of HIV have often forced seropositive people into the roles of victims or confessors of sexual guilt (Watney 1987).

As friends and lovers fell to the onslaught of the epidemic, gay men organized from the beginning into groups devoted to an ethic of caring for one another. Community-based organizations formed to spread the word about how to avoid HIV and to provide support to people with AIDS (Adam 1992c). Fresh from struggles against conservative offensives to roll back civil rights gains in the late 1970s and early 1980s, gay and lesbian activists regrouped to counter the effects of bureaucratic inertia and political budgeting priorities. AIDS activists, like Michael Callen, developed safer sex as an alternative to the "just say no" methods of prevention championed by the state and public health. AIDS activists fought for access to treatments and treatment information, supportive services, anonymous (as opposed to confidential) testing, and improved levels of research funding. They challenged the atmosphere of blame, bigotry, and inaction around AIDS and pressed forward a conception of health from below, emphasizing collective action to increase the power of those affected over their bodies and their lives (Sears 1991).[6] The context for making a life with HIV is therefore a contradictory one. The initial silences and reprobation contributed to shaping a poisonous atmosphere in which people living with HIV faced irrational fears of contagion, blame, and rejection. At the same time, the challenge of AIDS activism has created other possibilities, turning back stigma and clearing the ground for a "positive" identity.

The Participants

People live with HIV in a complex environment in which the attribution of stigma has been contested but certainly not defeated. Individuals may or may not have access to a way of living with HIV which challenges the epidemic of bigotry and blame that have accompanied AIDS. This access depends on geographic location, extent of integration into AIDS groups, and numerous other factors to be described below.

This work draws on interviews with 60 people with HIV disease or AIDS and 40 of their caregivers[7] living in southeastern Michigan and southwestern Ontario. They volunteered to be interviewed primarily through three routes: (1) following presentations made by the authors to support groups, (2) through personal referrals made by people who had already been interviewed, and (3) through other personal networks developed in AIDS-related organizations due to the authors' long-term involvement in community AIDS work. Gaining access to support groups typically involved meeting first with organization directors and then with individual group leaders. Group leaders then took our request to their groups; we visited only after having been invited by the group as a whole. Group members often examined us, sometimes very acutely, on a variety of issues including our personal connections to AIDS, the value and ethics of the study, and the benefits the study could have for them. The extended interaction of their granting permission to us in a collective decision-making forum, where they decided whether to participate as individuals, worked to create a level of informed consent well beyond that assured through the individual contract usually favored in research. The response was typically very good with majorities of each support group expressing willingness to participate.

This project differs from much of the established AIDS literature by drawing respondents from outside the epicenters of the epidemic[8] and by moving beyond the frequent concentration upon gay, white, male, and middle class subjects in order to follow the changing face of AIDS, as drug users, people of color, and women appear more frequently in the epidemiological statistics. Of seropositive respondents, 38 (63%) first mention a European ethnicity, 20 (33%) state they are black or African American, and two are aboriginal.[9] As well, two others next mention aboriginal ancestry and one, black ancestry in addition to the first-mentioned ethnicity. Thirty-four (57%) identify themselves as "gay" or "homosexual," 7 (12%) as bisexual, and 19 (32%) as heterosexual; 48 (80%) are men, 12, women; 35 (58%) are living on less than $10,000 per year, 24 on more. Finally, 15 (25%) mention having had infections which would qualify for the CDC Definition of AIDS, 35 (58%) mention symptoms consistent with HIV disease, and 10 (17%), no symptoms. Though we did not directly question study participants about drug use, 17 (28%) volunteered that they had gone through a drug rehabilitation program or had used intravenous drugs or cocaine with some frequency, 6 (10%) characterized themselves as alcoholic, and 4 spoke of "drinking a lot" or drinking "binges." Following are characteristics of study participants:

	Gay/bisexual men	Heterosexual men	Heterosexual women
White	31	4	4
Black	10	3	8

Given such a recruitment profile, no claim is presented here that this set of respondents fully represents the universe of seropositive people. It could be argued, for example, that people drawn from support groups may oversample those who have overcome the denial or fear which may inhibit their contact with an AIDS-related organization or, on the other hand, that they may undersample those who have "graduated" from support groups to coping particularly well on their own. Apart from the practical consideration that support groups offer one of the few locations where seropositive people can be easily found, support groups have the advantage of providing a relatively safe and comfortable site where potential participants could scrutinize us, question us (sometimes at length), and come to a well-informed decision about participation.

Apart from this demographic description, little enumeration or measurement of behavior appears in the following chapters. Rather, our approach is to chart the interactional linkages among everyday problems and the practical solutions which have been worked out in living with HIV disease. Each thematic section does report the more common responses first; less common, later, but at the same time, no attempt has been made here to collapse responses toward a mean or to cast away "outlier," singular, or unusual experiences. Indeed all of these experiences and practices have the potential to offer insight into the successful navigation of the treacherous currents of the "second illness" of "stigma, rejection, fear, and exclusion that attach to particularly dreaded disease" (Scheper-Hughes and Lock 1986:137). Respondents chose whether to be interviewed in their homes, our homes, or the site of their support groups. While we expressed a preference to interview people alone, their comfort was our primary concern. We interviewed all but four seropositive respondents individually. One was interviewed with a trusted caregiver and three friends were interviewed together in accordance with their preference. Forty-seven were interviewed in Michigan; 13 in Ontario. Interviews were conducted in 1990 and 1991 and typically lasted 1½ hours.

We started interviews with a series of conversation openers concerning areas of life potentially affected by HIV and found that participants had often already thought through their HIV-related experiences in the form of a coherent story. The interview schedule typically functioned as a trigger for this story which often unfolded in its entirety after three or four questions and required little further prompting by us.[10] We let participants define the issues most salient to them and allowed them to define the demographic categories reported above. It is important to note, for example, that some participants identified themselves as "heterosexual" after discussing lengthy personal histories of sex with people of their own sex; others identified themselves as "gay" while talking of their biological children. In talking about family, we asked about those whom participants most relied upon emotionally, financially, and practically (in terms of everyday, domestic assistance) and allowed them to specify the nature of the relationship and to name it as they saw fit. Rather than presuming any preexisting family form, participants talked of an array of friends, lovers, and fiancés in addition to more conventional kin terms. Our approach has been to preserve the participants' own terminology in describing themselves and to transcribe their speech without change or "correction." We later accessed interviews by means of the hypertext program, askSam.

The responses of the participants in this study are organized thematically rather than biographically, in that we show the various coping strategies employed to deal with HIV-related situations rather than viewing these strategies simply as the outcome of preexisting personality types. Phenomenological sociology does not presume a single coherent personality from which behavior flows, rather it looks for "recipe-knowledges" which can be drawn upon in dealing with particular situations. It does not impute consistency into people's activities but searches out the repertoire of recipes, projects, and strategies that can be used in social interaction. Our focus, then, is on coping strategies which are potentially available to anyone rather than embedding them in the peculiarities of the individuals who participated in this study.

We learned by listening to people with HIV a much more variegated geography of experience than prescribed by the current intellectual emphasis on difference and identity. Not long ago, social science methodology demanded adherence to an "objective," "universalist" viewpoint, a norm which concealed a reliance on a white male construction of the social world. The critique of this position has led to a particularism where people divided by gender, social class, race, and sexual orientation have often come to be treated as separate species of persons. The social location of people does vary by these characteristics, and those locations deeply shape the experiences of illness and its social consequences. At the same time, there are many times here that the commonality of experiences is striking and these different statuses have little to contribute to understanding how HIV disturbs everyday life. As well, these respondents challenge many of the conventional categories that have come to make up AIDS discourse. In these pages are: lesbian and transsexual caregivers to heterosexual women, gay male caregivers to heterosexual families, gay black professional men, and impoverished white gay men who defy glib generalizations about the social profile of people with HIV.

Gay communities in the epicenters of the epidemic, especially New York, San Francisco, and Toronto, rallied first to develop practical means of avoiding HIV transmission and to provide care for those who had become ill. Over time, a dense network of community-based institutions has come to extend support to HIV-positive people and their caregivers. A good deal of research has continued to focus on the epicenters. In this study, the participants come from communities where both the full impact of the epidemic and the response to it have come a few years later. Compared to the epicenters, there may be a higher proportion of gay men with HIV who move "back" to families of origin from major cities, and fewer who have weak or broken family ties along with strong alternative gay networks in the largest cities. Local gay community institutions tend not to be as extensive or well-developed as in the largest metropolises, which may affect the resources available to gay men with HIV in this study and the discourses they rely on for making sense of the syndrome. The study participants do reflect the growing diversity of communities affected by HIV. Women, African Americans, working class and unemployed people, rural people, and people with drug-using backgrounds articulate their experiences here in contrast to the many studies which have concentrated on more privileged informants. Indeed we have been surprised to find how little of the published work on women and AIDS has given voice to African American and drug using women, though these categories comprise *majorities* of women with AIDS in the United States. As Diane Lewis (1993:312) notes, "There have been few studies of African-American women intravenous (IV) drug-users' life experiences and self-perceptions (. . .), and virtually no published research on the impact of the AIDS epidemic on their outlook and behavior" (see also Hassin 1994). Finally, the binational character of this sample allows us unique insights into the effects of two very different national systems of medical care on the way HIV is experienced.

"Psycho-Social" Aspects

A look into the research literature on the "psycho-social aspects" of HIV and other life-threatening diseases reveals a preponderant number of studies done in hospitals and other clinical settings where the fundamental research concern turns out to be patient management or compliance. This clinical research typically concerns itself with the reasons why patients fail to take medication or rehabilitation regimes as prescribed by medical staff, and tends to make their behavior something mysterious and irrational by decontextualizing it from the nonclinical aspects of their lives. Much of the existing research literature points toward the conclusion that the predominant mode of studying people with AIDS, developed over the last fifteen years, is one of imposing pre-set measuring instruments upon them in order to arrive at conclusions that enhance the administrative power of professionals over their lives but that have little evident value for enabling seropositive people themselves.

So entrenched is this established model that funding agencies refuse studies which propose to take the words of seropositive people seriously, studies which use noncausal, qualitative methodologies, or studies which lead to understandings of direct use to HIV-positive people themselves. Such research often falls prey to the charge of lacking "scientificity" or "objectivity" for taking the subjectivity of AIDS seriously. These policies produce study after study which subject HIV-positive people to a battery of standardized psychometric tests which are then used, as for example in Diana Perkins et al. (1993), to impute "borderline personality disorder" and a grab-bag of other psychiatric labels to their ways of coping with stigmatized illness. In this instance, the authors then speculate about whether the supposed "personality disorder" of people with AIDS leads them to promiscuity and thus to exposure to HIV, or whether HIV disease leads to their "personality disorder"! Whether used to demonstrate elevated stress, anxiety, or depression (Atkinson et al. 1988; Joseph et al. 1990) or, as in this instance, "borderline personality disorder," the predominant research model strips away the sociopolitical environment in which people with HIV and their caregivers must live, suppresses the interactive processes through which they act in a hostile world, and makes their coping strategies irrational by removing the contexts which give them meaning (see Adam 1992b:4). The result is "knowledge" which further legitimates professional intervention in their lives but offers nothing to assist them in addressing the problems that concern them most (Clatts 1994:94). As Cindy Patton (1990b:53) observes:

> The knowledge that comes from the social and imaginary world—knowledge about surviving with a chronic illness, about reinventing sexual pleasure in a disaster zone, about finding the courage to transcend the narrowly defined roles of the AIDS service industry—these knowledges are either pushed to the margins of scientific knowledge or are rewritten as scientific data about odds of survival or aggregate behavior change.

Or as Juliet Corbin and Anselm Strauss (1988:xii) remark,

> little of this research [on chronic illness] has focused on the actual work of managing illness at home, and even less has examined the roles played by the partners of the chronically ill. In the course of our research, however, we have realized that the key players in the drama of accommodating chronic illness at home are the ill people and their spouses, rather than the assisting medical staff.

In the following chapters, the study participants talk of the ways in which they became aware of being HIV-positive, and their initial responses to the diagnosis. Because of the widespread identification of AIDS with particular "risk groups," people who identify themselves as members are often already alerted to the possibility of having contracted HIV. For others, such a diagnosis may be unexpected and occur as a result of institutional screening. Since the symptoms of HIV disease are highly variable and open to numerous interpretations, it is often not easy to determine what is related to HIV and what is not, even after having testing positive. Diagnosis with a life-threatening illness then raises a vast range of issues concerning the future, often within a context of feeling well. The process of identifying and coping with symptoms soon becomes a social undertaking as family, friends, physicians, and support groups offer opinions and advice concerning the meaning of the seropositive person's feelings. Out of these interactions emerge the strategies for coping with HIV both as a bodily and social disruption.

Making sense of HIV may then involve piecing together a number of discursive strands drawn from people in one's immediate environment. Institutions which propagate AIDS stories of their own may also affect

HIV-positive people so that pragmatic approaches may contend with religious or therapeutic constructions of what AIDS is "all about." The experience of illness is very much embedded in social contexts: social class,
gender, sexual orientation, and race all influence the resources and
understandings that can be brought to bear on making sense of HIV.

In chapters 4 and 5, participants discuss dilemmas raised in pursuing
new sexual and emotional relationships, as well as difficulties experienced by testing positive while in the midst of a current relationship.
While many fear their sexual lives have been irrevocably spoiled, others
find, through trial and error, new possibilities. Families have the potential to be either one of the greatest sources of support or one of the
biggest problems to deal with. Strategies for disclosing HIV status to
family members often include identifying who is likely to be empathetic
or judgmental, deciding what can be said to children, figuring out how
to discuss homosexual or drug-using practices, and feeling out friends
and in-laws.

Having HIV and going to work raises another realm of issues that
needs solutions. Those who are ill may need to appeal to the good will
of their employers so that they can compensate for their illness with time
off or different duties. Employers, all too frequently, jump to the conclusion that HIV is incompatible with staying at work even when employees are well and entirely capable of continuing on the job. Human rights
legislation has had very limited effectiveness in protecting the participants in this study from discrimination. Where medical insurance is
work-related, losing a job may have far-reaching consequences just at the
point when a person most needs good medical attention. By interviewing people in a country with universal medical coverage (Canada) and a
country with private coverage (United States), it is possible to discern
the effects of the overall social organization of medical services on the
experiences of people in medical need.

EXPERIENCING HIV

Chapter One

IN THE BEGINNING

The diagnosis of being HIV-positive opens a new and difficult journey of restabilizing a life jarred from its foundations. People come to be tested for HIV antibodies in very different circumstances and draw on a wide range of meanings and resources to meet the challenge of a life-threatening illness. At one end of a spectrum are those who virtually diagnose themselves through assessing symptoms in light of personal histories of risk activity. This occurs more often in situations where individuals know others who are HIV-positive or are members of a community with a high level of knowledge about AIDS. In these instances, the test confirms (or contradicts) a suspected diagnosis. Others, by contrast, begin to think of themselves as being at risk for HIV only through the process of being tested. This includes people tested while under medical care for a health problem or through screening programs. This chapter explores the ways in which HIV is discovered and then handled.

Among the participants in this study, it was primarily gay men who sought out testing after identifying themselves as being at risk for HIV infection. Popular conceptions of AIDS, reinforced by both the mainstream and the gay press, as well as community-based AIDS organizations, have strongly associated homosexuality with AIDS, allowing few gay-identified men able to feel secure that they have escaped the virus. Still, this awareness is far from uniform even among men with homosexual interests. Men who have sex with men who do not identify as gay very often lack contact with the gay community and its information networks, or exclude themselves, like many heterosexual men, from the category of being "at risk." (The relationship between homosexual behavior and gay identity is explored further in chapter 3.) Outside of the gay male population, access to AIDS information and awareness of risk declines appreciably, particularly among women, people of color, and those with lower education or income. People who have less awareness of personal risk are more likely to be tested after developing symptoms, through screening programs, or as a result of some precipitating event such as the infection of a friend or lover.

Since 1985, the technical process of diagnosis for HIV infection has been relatively simple, consisting of a blood test to identify antibodies to the virus, but the social process may be much more complex. Popular misconceptions tend to associate a positive diagnosis with a "death sentence." This "common sense" knowledge may prove quite resilient, both among those who test positive and their families, friends, and lovers. The already serious implications of an HIV-positive diagnosis are thus likely to be exaggerated in the perception of those receiving the news. Not only do the (real or exaggerated) health issues associated with an HIV-positive diagnosis make it difficult to receive test results, but many people also anticipate the stigma often associated with HIV infection. The social prognosis may seem as problematic as the medical one.

Fear of potentially devastating social consequences has made many people reluctant to seek testing. The guarantee of anonymity has, over time, emerged as a widespread public health policy in order to encourage people to find out their health status. The availability of anonymous testing figures prominently in some people's decisions about getting tested. As Paula,[1] a full-time mother living on government assistance, remarked:

> I am one of those persons—as long as it is anonymous testing and they don't ask questions I go, so that is how I found out. (heterosexual black female)

Having an HIV test done at a doctor's office is protected by the confidentiality governing all medical records, but it is far from anonymous. Confidential testing means that an individual's name is attached to the result and may be reported to public health officials, insurance providers, or other medical personnel. Doctors may be less aware of how tenuous confidentiality is in this situation than the people whose lives are at stake. Wayne, a computer worker in his thirties, relates this incident:

> The emergency doctor—I didn't know him from anywhere—and he sat me down, and he gave me the results. . . . He said "confidential" and everything, but then he opened his door, and said, "Here I want a copy of this." (gay white male)

Just as Scambler (1984:216) found that the stigma associated with epilepsy leads to a "predisposition to secrecy," there is a very real need with HIV disease to contain information that can have consequences in employment, family relationships, insurance, and other issues. Ultimately, anonymous testing protects only the sero-status of those who test negative. For those who test positive, entry into medical treatment, application for drugs paid for by governments, and legal requirements that positive tests be reported to public health authorities mean that they have to rely on the practices of numerous medical workers to preserve confidentiality.

The testing process is therefore freighted with real and exaggerated health concerns, fears about stigma, and apprehensions about control over information. Testing has an intensity that sets this moment in high relief, and can influence the first steps taken toward rebuilding a life now inseparable from HIV.

Testing Without Symptoms

Diagnosis follows the development of symptoms for most medical conditions. The diagnosis of HIV infection in the absence of symptoms occurs in one of three ways: First, some people seek out voluntary testing as the result of an assessment of their risk activities. Second, people who have no symptoms may be diagnosed as HIV-positive through mandatory tests that are required in certain situations in the United States such as imprisonment, military enlistment, or immigration. Third, people may be identified as HIV-positive through screening programs such as those aimed at protecting the blood supply.

The incidence of asymptomatic testing likely increased substantially when effective medical treatments became available and, as a consequence, AIDS organizations began recommending it in the late 1980s. In the midst of the public panic of the mid-1980s, when little was known about the course of the disease and there was little effective treatment of opportunistic infections, it seemed pointless to seek out the test. Indeed at a time when anonymous testing sites were scarce, the dangerous social consequences of testing HIV-positive seemed to outweigh any benefits which could come from seeking medical treatment. As treatment improved and much of the public panic dissipated, the position of AIDS organizations shifted in the late 1980s. Asymptomatic testing came to be promoted for people at risk so they could seek early treatment and make lifestyle changes useful for improving their well-being. Testing became part of a process of seeking out information in order to take control over one's own health (Levine and Bayer 1989).

It was primarily gay men in this study who voluntarily sought testing in the absence of symptoms. The participants in this study, then, reflect the pattern identified by Lynn Paringer, Kathryn Phillips, and Teh-wei Hu (1991:230–34), where "risk group" membership best predicts voluntary testing. They also found that men were more likely to be tested than women, even when controlling for "risk group" membership. The likelihood of seeking out testing increased with education but decreased with family income. Young people, blacks, and people who were well informed about AIDS were more likely to seek out testing than others.

Gay men in this study most often considered themselves at risk and had the access to resources necessary for testing. Andy was tested at a time when the issue was very current among his peers. As he remarked, "Testing was in the air." Steve, a florist in his forties, was tested at the same time as many of his friends, spurred on by optimism connected to the introduction of AZT:

> Well actually everybody was getting the test. . . . AZT came out I believe at that time, so I said, I was under the impression that it was something that was a cure at the time. (gay white male)

Some gay men are tested on a regular basis. Jeff, a nurse in his twenties, started such a routine after assessing the riskiness of his sexual activities:

> I had been getting myself tested over a period of a year and a half every three to four months on the basis of knowing my own sexual history and my own health. (gay aboriginal and white male)

Jordan, a salesman in his twenties, developed a similar routine after an incident that made him aware of his risk.

> See I had a little scare about a year and a half before I was diagnosed so I went ahead and got the full testing and it was negative. Due to the kind of sexual lifestyle I was leading, I will always have a scare. It became to be more or less habit. I would try to get myself tested every 6 months. (bisexual black male)

While the awareness of risk led some people to get themselves tested, others avoided testing because of fears associated with that very awareness. Some people felt they should be tested but avoided it until they faced problems with their health. Peter, a salesman in his forties, waited for two years to get tested.

> I thought, well, I should be tested and then I started having some real health problems and that went on for about two years, went back and forth. (gay white male)

Dan, a waiter in his thirties, decided not to be tested despite his awareness of risk. There seemed to be a lot of potential pain and no real benefits in knowing his HIV status in the mid-1980s when less was known about treatment and prevention.

> I didn't see what would be positive about getting the test taken. There were less things on the positive side of getting that test taken because I didn't know what you could do about it. So you are positive, what do you do? What advantage does that give you? (gay white male)

He eventually decided to get tested but chose not to go back for the results. The period between getting tested and hearing the results can be particularly trying.

> I don't know what made me go in for the test. I had some friends who were taking it. And I didn't go back for the results. I talked to them and they did some counselling . . . and they called me back and they said to come back in and I don't know why, but at that time I couldn't handle it. I just didn't go back in.

AIDS, then, has an immediacy for large numbers of gay men that leads some to be tested on a voluntary basis without any symptoms. This immediacy derives both from the overall level of AIDS education in the community and the proximity of friends' experiences with testing and HIV infection. This same immediacy leads others to avoid testing at times when they feel unable to deal with the consequences.

Like some gay men, heterosexual people also go for the test when HIV enters their lives through an event that flags the possibility of HIV infection. Paula was prompted to get tested during pregnancy by the illness of her boyfriend, which in the end was not HIV-related. She did not expect an antibody-positive test result as she had neither symptoms nor a history of what she defined as risk activities.

I don't have any of the symptoms. I wasn't an alcohol user. I wasn't a
drug abuser, so I figured I was straight 'til the test came back. No, I was
HIV positive. (heterosexual black female)

News reports brought home the risk associated with injection drug use
to Shadonna.

I would hear about it on the news and I kept hearing "AIDS." . . . I kept
listening to them and they kept saying, "gay men and IV drug users."
. . . So I told my doctor, I said, . . . "Do you take the AIDS test here?" I
thought that I could have it because I am a recovering addict from IV
drug use. (heterosexual black female)

Lemuel, a cook in his forties, got tested after another patient at a drug
treatment facility raised the issue of risk for AIDS. He had previously considered his risk activities through sex with other men, but "didn't want
to face up to it."

I was . . . on the substance abuse ward, and this guy came in there,
young white guy, very intelligent, and the rest of the guys up there
were like, hard core junkies. . . . And he kept saying, "Everyone up
here should be tested for AIDS." . . . And he was saying, "Well I am
going to get tested. What about you, Lemuel?" And so I told him, "Oh
sure, yeah" although I was scared to death. (gay black male)

Some people found themselves quite suddenly confronted with HIV
testing as a result of the condition of a partner or child. Nick, a biolo-
gist in his forties, got tested after his partner was surprised by an HIV-
positive diagnosis.

[I]t was a result of him being tested. The issue of being tested never
entered my mind. He was tested when he was in the hospital for
another issue, another reason, and just said, "Do it." But when it came
back, the result, I automatically tested myself, had myself tested. . . .
There was no prior knowledge or even consideration. (gay white male)

Similarly, Andrea, a secretary in her thirties, got tested "because my
fiancé was tested. He was tested positive . . . so that is why I got tested."
The seropositivity of a sex partner may suddenly confront people with
their own risk for HIV infection. The same thing can happen through the
testing of recently born child. Luelle became aware of her HIV status
through the testing of her son.

I didn't [get tested myself]. I had my son and they tested him. . . . I
went home first and they kept him three days. After I went home and

when they told me to come and pick him up, that's when they told me. (heterosexual black female)

Finding Out Through Institutional Procedures

Others were tested as part of routine institutional procedures whether they were experiencing symptoms or not. Institutional testing typically occurs in situations where people lack many of the usual legal defenses against official intrusion: e.g., when they are prisoners, soldiers, patients, or immigrants. Three participants in this study were diagnosed as HIV-positive through mandatory testing in prisons or the armed forces. Jim, a student in his twenties, was tested in prison in Michigan. He said that he had not been informed that his blood would be tested for HIV.

> No, they just do it. It is mandatory since 1989; they made it in federal and state [prisons that they] test all the inmates before they are released now. (bisexual black male)

Mike was tested soon after his arrival in prison. Although a prison doctor gave him a card with a number to call, he did not feel comfortable following it up. He spent his term dealing with the positive test result in fear for his safety and without support. Like other prison inmates, Mike kept his HIV status quiet for fear of developing a "bad reputation."

> But I be seeing some guys in prison, I knew they had it. But . . . they be trying to make it stay as far away from them as possible. If you say some bad thing, bad reputation would get around. (heterosexual black male)

Joe, a teacher in his twenties, was discharged after the Navy tested him as a result of the mandatory testing policy of the United States military. Although he had previously been tested when he was ill, those results had been negative.

> The first time I was tested I was sick. I had reason to suspect that I was positive. The first test, I was negative. Second and third test, I was negative. So then like the fourth test that I was doing for a job situation, to go into an officer's program with the navy, that's when there was a positive. . . . I was discharged immediately. (bisexual black male)

Mandatory testing generally confronts people with HIV-positive results without adequate preparation or support resources, making their adjustment especially difficult. It also exposes them to potential or actual discrimination because the test results are known to authorities with power over them. Joe was offered helpful counselling through individuals in the Navy, while neither Mike nor Jim received much support in prison.

Along with mandatory testing, some people are diagnosed as the result of screening programs with particular goals. One couple learned of their HIV-status after the introduction of a program to screen hemophiliacs and their partners. Others were identified through the screening program which tests donated blood in order to protect the blood supply. Barb and Gordon were tested as part of a study in 1985 to identify the prevalence of HIV among hemophiliacs and their partners. The testing was done at a time when the general level of AIDS education was low and few people knew of the high rate of infection among hemophiliacs and their partners. Barb did not recall making an informed choice to be tested.

> We didn't decide we were going to be tested. We didn't decide to. We didn't know what we were being tested for. . . . The testing issue, really didn't exist like it does for people now, that have to decide whether or not they want to know. (heterosexual white and aboriginal female)

Her partner, Gordon, said that he had understood the purpose of the test and went ahead on the assumption that they would test negative.

> We had heard, to be honest . . . that the AIDS virus had found its way into the blood supply, but we didn't know anybody first hand who was feeling any ill effects. So I guess we just said, it could be, but there are a lot of things that could be. If we go in and have this test it is probably going to be negative. Why don't we just take it? (heterosexual white male)

With so little known about the prognosis for people who tested positive, Barb and Gordon were devastated by the result.

> They [medical personnel] clearly just said, "We don't understand what this means. It means you have been, we know you have been exposed to it. Now it can never bother you the rest of your life, you could be sick in 5 years, you could be sick and dead in 5 weeks. We have absolutely nothing to go by at this point. (heterosexual white male)

The screening of blood donations also turns up asymptomatic individuals who test antibody positive. Three of the participants in this study were regular blood donors who had not anticipated that they might be HIV positive. This proved particularly shocking to Alex, a 41-year-old prison worker, who was informed of his diagnosis through the mail without counselling.

> I used to give [at] blood drives. . . . So the one particular time in July of '87, I gave at a blood drive. . . . about three weeks later I get a registered letter. I read it. It said I had HIV and they recommended I go see a doctor. (bisexual black male)

The two others, who discovered their HIV status through making blood donations, had donated blood as an indirect way of being tested for HIV. Daniel, a motel worker in his twenties, found that this was not a good way to get tested as he was not offered adequate counselling.

> I didn't know anything about HIV testing and I was kind of afraid to get tested and everything and so I said, "Well, I've always given blood in the past so I'll just go give blood and if they—." I know it's a bad way to do it, but that's what I did—and, wow, two months have gone by, this is great, three months have gone by, it must be negative. And then I was at work one day and I got a phone call from the guy I was living with. He said, "Daniel, a registered letter from the Health Unit just came in." I said, "Go ahead and open it." He told me right over the phone. (gay white male)

While this testing route is strongly discouraged by AIDS organizations as it poses a risk to the blood supply, blood screening may still turn up HIV among the unsuspecting and among those who resist making a fully conscious choice to ascertain their sero-status.

Sorting Out Symptoms

Despite the general availability of the HIV-antibody test and better public understanding about risk factors, many people still find out only as a result of falling ill and receiving a medical diagnosis. In the beginning of the epidemic, before the test and at a time when the transmission and identification of the syndrome were not well understood, only people with serious illness could be diagnosed. The introduction of the HIV antibody test in 1985, combined with the development of screening programs and mandatory testing in specific situations, opened the possibility of early diagnosis of HIV disease. Nonetheless, many people are not diagnosed until they are ill. People who do not consider themselves at risk for HIV, those who have not been reached by adequate AIDS education, and people who do not have access to medical services, particularly in the United States, are not likely to seek out voluntary testing when they have no symptoms. Research on women and HIV infection shows that women tend to be diagnosed later in their infection than men, often in response to some precipitating event such as the testing of one of their children (Hunter 1995:36; Bury 1994:19). In this study, women, people of color, and people with lower incomes more often tested once they are symptomatic. At the same time, some white gay men also tested only after the onset of illness. The prospect of facing a life-threatening illness deters many from finding out, and the early symptoms of HIV disease are ambiguous enough to be attributed to other causes. As well, some people found they had been tested for HIV in hospitals or drug rehabilitation centers when they were seeking help for medical conditions unrelated to HIV. This section explores the process by which the signs of physical disorder come to be read as HIV disease.

The decision to be tested may follow a period of self assessment where lingering suspicions cohere into a strong sense that symptoms "add up" to HIV disease. Peter figured it out this way:

> I started having some real memory disfunction and short term memory loss, real severe. I was getting lost on street corners in a town I had lived in all my life. I'd be a block from my house and have no idea where I was at. . . . I was totally lost. And so I went to the doctor . . . In the process, I asked him at the time maybe we should consider, you know, the HIV test and he said, "Well, it's a possibility." (gay white male)

In some instances, HIV disease is identified as the consequence of a medical crisis. Lemuel was tested after going to a hospital for urgent medical attention.

> I got sick so I had to go to emergency. While I was in emergency they were trying to find out as well. They had found that I had tuberculosis. So along with the tuberculosis, they found that I was past the stage of HIV. I had ARC.[2] (gay black male)

Robbie, a teacher in his forties, went into hospital with pneumonia. His doctor suggested an HIV test.

> As soon as the doctor found out that I was gay, he asked me if I wanted to be tested. I was panicking and I said, "Sure" and that was that. (gay white male)

Medical emergencies often create feelings of lack of control and anxiety which can easily be exacerbated by an HIV-positive diagnosis. They can also create a situation in which HIV testing is embarked on with little forethought as part of an ongoing medical intervention. Ron, a com-

puter analyst in his twenties, asked his doctor to add an HIV test to the
others he was performing to diagnose swollen tonsils.

> I did it basically on a whim. One night I woke up and my tonsils were
> swollen, totally unrelated to the HIV but while I was at the doctor's I
> said, "Well throw in an HIV [test] anyway." (gay white male)

The addition of one more test might seem relatively minor at a moment
when medical intrusions are already under way. Gregory, a sales clerk in
his twenties, took an HIV test at the clinic that he went to for the diagnosis and treatment of another sexually transmitted disease. He accepted
the additional test quite casually, as he had not expected it would come
out positive.

> When I got tested, I went to a VD clinic in Toronto and they just asked
> me if I wanted to get the AIDS antibody test and I said, "Sure." I didn't
> think it was going to happen or anything, so I went to this clinic and
> they tested me there. (gay white male)

The casual addition of an HIV test to an ongoing medical intervention
may result in pre-test counselling and informed consent being shortened
or passed over altogether. A number of participants mentioned that they
were tested without giving informed consent. Crystal said that she had not
been informed that her blood was being tested for HIV during pregnancy.

> I didn't know they were taking those tests. You know they take your blood
> every so often when you are pregnant. (heterosexual black female)

While it is possible that medical personnel did obtain what they understood to be informed consent, a patient who is undergoing a battery of
tests in a highly vulnerable moment might consent to an additional procedure without fully understanding it. Alternatively, regulations requiring informed consent may not be observed at all. That was certainly the
perception of Camillo, who reported:

> I was scheduled to have an operation and they tested my blood. . . .
> The doctor refused to operate. . . . I had no counselling; was handed
> a couple of pamphlets and that was it. (heterosexual white male)

Richard, a thirty-seven year old man now living on government assistance, discovered that his doctor had used indirect methods to find indi-
cators of HIV infection without informing him.

> In my situation I was sort of tricked into it. . . . After I got out of the
> hospital, my doctor sent me for blood tests and I wasn't going to go for

them, but the person I was seeing at the time said, "Well, go for them," and well what he was doing, he was doing my T4s. . . . In November '87 when they found my T4s were 300, that's when he sat down and talked to me. (gay white male)

Drug rehabilitation programs may also include HIV testing among a series of interventions without their clients being fully cognizant of it. Two participants mentioned that they were tested without informed consent while in treatment centers. Rick was tested in a drug rehabilitation center "without my knowledge." (His initial diagnosis is discussed below.) Ninia, a housewife and former sex worker, described a similar experience of being tested without fully understanding or consenting.

I'll tell you the first three times I was tested, I don't ever remember signing anything. Nobody asked me the first time I was pregnant. I was also addicted to heroin. I went into a Methadone clinic for pregnant women and the next thing I knew, the counselor wanted to talk to me and he told me I had AIDS. He suggested I get with God. (heterosexual white female)

People tested while seeking treatment of other medical conditions often find themselves confronted with a situation for which they are not prepared. Rhonda, a medical assistant in her twenties, was tested on her doctor's advice without much thought as she assumed that she would test negative.

I was pregnant and I was going to my regular OB doctor and I had told him that I had been having some really bad lower pains. Usually when you have female problems, they ask that you be tested and so I thought, "OK, no problem, because I am not going to have HIV." (heterosexual white female)

The combination of an HIV-positive diagnosis with other health problems can create a particularly traumatic entry into life with HIV infection. This diagnosis may be a completely unexpected complication to an already difficult situation.

Being Told

Hearing an HIV-positive test result challenges many of the most fundamental assumptions about how one's life is expected to unfold. The hallmark of anticipating a life with HIV, or many other chronic illnesses, is uncertainty (Weitz 1989, Bury 1982). Many of the landmarks which give order to one's life may suddenly lose their solidity as the uncertain trajectory of infection raises such issues as dependence on others, increased reliance on the medical system, disability, and death. Testing positive explodes many of the stories we tell ourselves about who we are, where we are going, and what other people think of us. As the painful inadequacy of one's taken-for-granted routines and habits comes to the fore, a search begins to assimilate the unwelcome news, sort out its implications, and reorder a life made fragile and uncertain. Professionals responsible for notifying people of their test results often provide the initial advice on reorganizing a life vulnerable to the disruption of HIV. This section explores the experience of being told, and first efforts to make sense of life in a more treacherous universe. For Fred, an unemployed social worker, testing positive felt like this:

> And it was like for a fraction of a second everything stopped in my body. I went numb, totally numb. . . . He said HIV was just the germ of the AIDS virus, and that I could probably get hit by a bus or a car, and die from that, before I die from this. But it was like he was talking and I was there, and it was like cloudy, my body was there but my head was somewhere else, and there was no tears. I had no emotions, I just sat there. (gay black male)

What is most helpful is some combination of medical information with a discussion of social aspects of life with HIV which presents possibilities for life in the future. Many participants were offered neither the information nor the sense of hope that might have helped them in their transition to seropositivity. It is not surprising, given the character of the widespread media coverage about AIDS, that many people associate HIV infection with imminent death. Rather than uncertainty, many people begin their life with HIV in a state of misguided certainty. Gregory got very little from his doctor.

> He didn't explain nothing in detail. He actually made me think that I was going to die quickly, the way he explained it. (gay white male)

A prison doctor was similarly uninformative when giving Kevin, who was an inmate at the time, the results of his mandatory HIV test.

> Then they had one lady, a psychiatric counselor, that could give you information on the disease. She didn't have much information, just some brochures, and the doctor at the particular institution that I was at, he didn't know anything about the disease. He just told me the test

was positive and you are going to die and I don't know much about it.
(heterosexual black male)

Bill, a well-educated man now living on government assistance, described
a good counselling experience as one which conveyed a sense of hope.
He got this only after "firing" his previous doctor, who offered neither
optimism nor adequate information.

> That particular doctor. . . . was very much more helpful then the first
> doctor. He didn't say it was a death sentence. "There are a lot of med-
> icines out. You can live a long life if you don't give up your dreams."
> (gay black male)

Fred was pleased with the counselling he received at an AIDS organization. He was offered a number of services and introduced to programs
he required.

> Her thing was to expose me to people that could answer these ques-
> tions, because she was doing her job, finding me a place, making sure
> I was getting settled. She sent me applications for SSI [social assis-
> tance], section 8 [housing], for my half fare [transportation]. She was
> doing everything. She helped me get my furniture, original furniture,
> so then she told me about doctors that I could go to and she thought
> I should see a therapist. She said she was scared that once it was going
> to hit me, so I am seeing a therapist now. (gay black male)

One of the key pieces of medical information that might help people
with their transition is a discussion of the distinction between HIV infection and AIDS. Marcia did not get even this basic information.

> They didn't tell me anything about HIV infection. They just told me I
> had AIDS. (heterosexual black female)

Philip, an office manager in his thirties, had prepared for his test results
by doing some reading about HIV infection. The person who gave him
his test results at a clinic, however, offered up inaccuracies which shook
his confidence in the research he had done.

> She was just very, very rude. I said, "Well that means I tested positive for
> HIV," and she said, "No, this means you have AIDS." I read this brochure
> and I had gone over it before the test and it said very specifically in there,
> but she disagreed with the brochure and at that point she is an author-
> ity figure and I am not in a state to really defend myself, so I thought,
> "Oh my God I have AIDS," which I don't. (heterosexual white male)

Accurate medical information cannot eliminate the uncertainties that surround the transition to life with HIV. It can, however, contribute to eliminating the misguided certainties of imminent death and provide some perspective on possibilities for the future. Of course, the uncertainty that faces people living with HIV or other chronic illnesses does not only revolve around medical issues. Bury (1988:90) states that people are generally unaware in advance of the "limits of tolerance" others in their social circles will bring to the issues an illness may raise.

There are a number of specifically social issues surrounding life with HIV that may not be touched upon in initial counselling. Scambler (1984:225) reports that many of the people with epilepsy in his study were upset that doctors concentrated on conveying medical information and had little to say about, "personal adjustment and adaptation." This fits with the experience of a number of people in this study. Perhaps the extreme case is Gregory, who was given this information about the social aspects of living with HIV.

> But I didn't get any pretest or post-test counselling. One doctor said, well once I tested positive he said, "Well you are not allowed to have sex any more. The only thing you can do is masturbate." (gay white male)

The counselling that accompanies diagnosis has generally improved since the early years of AIDS. Gordon, a computer analyst in his thirties, described his experience of testing positive in the mid-1980s which combined maximum trauma with minimal useful information.

> [The] physician came in along with a couple of the nurses and said, "You tested positive" and they sort of sat at the opposite end of the room, as small as it was, and it was, "Gee these people are going to die before they get out of the room." I mean that was the kind of expression. (heterosexual white male)

He connected the lack of information with his experience of being diagnosed early in the epidemic.

> The pioneers definitely live with arrows in their backs, but I guess somebody has got to be first.

Some people received their diagnosis in situations where it was impossible to work through uncertainty by genuinely discussing their situation. Marcia, an unemployed medical worker, was given her test results in a room filled with doctors.

I have been off of drugs for about six years. I got sick. I was pregnant, six months pregnant and I got really sick and I had to go into the hospital. They admitted me in for pneumonia and while I was there they asked if I wanted to be tested for HIV infection and I told them, "Yea go ahead." About fifteen doctors came back to my room, about a week later. Fifteen doctors came back to my room. "Know that test that you consented to take?" and I said, "Yea." I said, "Oh no, I have AIDS," and one of the doctors said, "Yea." I was just scared to death when they told me. (heterosexual black female)

Rick, a thirty-three year old man now working as an AIDS educator, was told he tested positive for HIV when he returned to a drug treatment center for a Christmas party. He was planning to leave town the next day and the doctor had very little choice. The net effect, however, was to leave him in a situation where it was very difficult to deal with the information.

I was at a Christmas party when I was told [by a physician]. . . . he just told me there. So I had to go back out afterwards to this group of people . . . knowing nothing about the disease . . . no pre-test counselling, no post-test counselling. I didn't get nothing. (heterosexual white male)

A few people received their diagnosis over the phone. This left them without any real support at an extremely difficult moment. Dan was informed in this way.

I got it [test results] over the phone. The secretary gave me the results very coldly, just gave them to me. It didn't bother me at that point, because I already thought that they were positive. (gay white male)

Jason, a payroll clerk in his fifties, was informed of his test results over the phone at work. Even though the doctor at the other end of the line was quite sensitive, this left him in an impossible situation.

So we did the HIV test through my gastroenterologist. She called me at work and gave me my results over the phone. She was very compassionate, very considerate. She was wonderful except it was done there at my desk. I'm at work. It was very rough to maintain my composure for the rest of the day. (gay white male)

Post-test counselling can, at best, offer only momentary assistance. Gregory wanted to see a friend right away but had not arranged anything in advance.

After I got my results back I went and seen a friend. At first there was nobody home, like when I went there, so I sat at the apartment and I cried, and I kept on saying, "Why me?" and looked up at the sky. And I waited, and I waited, and I wanted somebody to talk to, but I didn't know hardly anybody there. (gay white male)

Carrying On

Testing positive poses what Bury (1982:169–70) describes as a "biographical disruption." In response, people mobilize various resources to reorganize their lives and belief systems. People proceed, in very different ways, to act on their new situation. Some change their lives very little, carrying on much as they had before. Others experience a wrenching shock that leaves them unable to continue, though this feeling often passes. Some are pushed by this crisis to take more control over their lives and achieve new goals.

Especially for those without symptoms, the results of an HIV test may seem entirely "unreal" and disconnected from their everyday experiences. Some respondents, especially those influenced by drug and alcohol recovery programs, describe carrying on much as before as being in "denial." Yet as Kathy Charmaz (1991:16–17) remarks, describing this coping pattern as "denial" presumes an "appropriate" response to illness when "carrying on" may be as successful as any other strategy. Joy, a 41-year-old woman in a job training program, described her response to testing positive this way:

> But the guy, where I had the testing done at, he sat down and he talked to me, told he about a program that I can get myself involved in. But I have never contacted any of them because I just go about my business like I always do. (bisexual black female)

Barb noted that when she was diagnosed in 1985 there was little that could be done. Carrying on with life seemed to be the most sensible option.

> At that time what there was to know was that it was a death sentence, that was all that they knew, and there was no drugs or anything like that. The therapies, like I said, there was no advantage to knowing then, like there is now. . . . So we just decided that I guess we will pretend that it just didn't happen, we just won't think about it, and we won't do anything for or against or whatever, just carried on the way it was. (heterosexual white and aboriginal female)

Another way of carrying on with life is to continue with the plans and goals that preceded diagnosis. Paula felt her plans for the future had not

changed. She had always concentrated on parenting and could continue
to do so.

> My plans didn't change at all, because I like to stay at home. I went to
> college. I could get a good job, at least $10 an hour, if I wanted to go
> to work, but when I was growing up my mother was gone all the time,
> so I decided in my life, when I had kids I was going to stay at home and
> be a ma. So my plans didn't change at all. (heterosexual black female)

Carrying on can also be linked to a sense of fatalism but Rhonda also
faced doubts that she would not see her plans through.

> Just like little things went through my mind, like "Am I still going to
> see my 2 year old graduate?" Things like that, but no particular plans
> have changed. I still want to be a nurse. I still want to send my daugh-
> ter through college. Everything is staying the same because I could go
> out on the street and get hit by a bus tomorrow and it could end, so.
> Sometimes they slip. Should I make these plans if I am not going to be
> here to go through with it? (heterosexual white female)

Ninia now considers her initial response to have been an instance of
denial. She was pregnant when she was tested and dismissed the result
because her partner had tested negative.

> So here I was facing pregnancy and this guy was telling me I had
> AIDS. The baby, the chances of going through withdrawal, it was
> quite a day. And I went in complete denial when they told me this,
> because my husband is still negative, as a matter of fact, so he would
> get tested and he was negative. It was easy for us to say, "Well they
> made a mistake," so it was easy for us to go into denial. (heterosex-
> ual white female)

Sheila, a former waitress now living on a disability pension, simply did
not digest the positive test result when it was given to her.

> I got tested. I was positive. I was using coke at the time too, so I didn't
> really care, like I didn't want to do anything about it. I was scared and
> all that. . . . And when I got straight I thought I had a lot of stomach
> problems, I was really sick, so I decided after I got out of that recovery
> home, to go get tested again, and I did and that is when I found out I
> was. (heterosexual white female)

Carrying on may be a strategy which is hard to sustain as events occur
which bring home the threat posed by HIV disease. Gordon found his
sense of normality overlaid a larger feeling of anxiety.

I realized that I just put it away in the back of my mind, but it was bothering me at a low level. As we knew more people that were becoming ill, it was becoming harder and harder to deny that it could be you. (heterosexual white male)

Carrying on as before may work as a form of avoidance of unresolved problems. Fred broke up with his partner and moved away to another city, moving relatively rapidly from a professional job in one city to living in a housing project for the homeless in another. It was there that he started to seek help.

I don't feel good about having this, but I do feel good taking the initiative to want to do something about it and I found out the more I tried to help myself, the more people tried to help me. (gay black male)

Shock and Reorientation

Even those who expect a sero-positive diagnosis at some level may feel that nothing could adequately prepare them for the shock. Despite his substantial experience with AIDS issues, Brad, a former nurse, reported:

I work for the health department doing the AIDS testing. I was doing the counselling for others and yet I was blown away by my diagnosis. (gay white male)

Philip was disoriented by his diagnosis even though he had expected it.

I really didn't do much of anything for a couple weeks. I was really in shock. Even though I knew ahead of time that it was going to be positive, it was still a shock. (gay white male)

This initial shock and dislocation may be accompanied by a sharp sense of anger. This is the way Camillo reacted.

The first symptoms I got were psychological. . . . I started getting very, very angry. Real angry. Angry at everybody and everything and I had an absolutely horrible attitude and it was uncharacteristic. . . . and I didn't know where this came from. (heterosexual white male)

The experience of shock is bound to be particularly intense if the diagnosis is associated with imminent death. People who do not already have considerable knowledge about HIV infection and AIDS are likely to summon this up as their first response to testing. Paula summed up her knowledge of AIDS at the time of diagnosis in the following words, "All I knew was you get AIDS and you are dead. That is all I knew." The association between a positive HIV test result and death can be particularly strong among people who are seriously ill when diagnosed. Robbie described these associations as well as the feeling of being given a "second chance" when he survived.

> The first time [I was tested] I was a mess because I was in the hospital all alone. I had no diagnosis of what was wrong with me, other than it was pneumonia. I thought I was dying. I thought it was the worst, it was the final phase of AIDS. I was gone and I was dying, and crying a lot and making peace with myself about the whole thing, so that when those three or four days were over I think I had come to grips with an awful lot of stuff, and then realized that, well at that point I thought there was nothing wrong. It was like being given a second chance. (gay white male)

Part of the initial shock may be the collapse of one's sense of the future. Aspirations and expectations, perhaps not even consciously held, may make themselves felt through their sudden disappearance. A new sense of mortality threatens long-term projects and deferred dreams, forcing a reconsideration of their viability. Some of the revaluation of the future may go too far as it is based on a belief that death is just around the corner. Indeed several participants in this study regretted giving up their plans as they adjusted to their HIV status and found that they continued to live in good health years after their diagnosis. Joe's plans changed abruptly as he had to leave the armed forces because of his HIV status. He found himself in a situation which he described as "in limbo," where his old plans were no longer possible but new plans were limited by an uncertain future.

> My plans changed because . . . now I was stuck with a 4 year empty calender. What do I do now? I would have liked to have gone somewhere else, back to school perhaps, rather then come home, but by not being totally sure of being just HIV positive, not being full blown, and not being negative either there was a limbo situation, pretty uncomfortable for me. That uncertainty was an emotional drain to say the least, and it was like carrying a baggage, so if I had some certainty and knew what I could plan for, I would have made alternative plans. I would have gone to enhance my life in another ways. (bisexual black male)

Bob (who had become an AIDS activist) continued with his short-term plans but lost his longer range perspective.

Well, you give up your long-term twenty and thirty year plans. . . . I haven't lost my two and three year plans. I still plan a year down the road, a year and a half, two years. Still planning that year or two keeps pushing, keeps you going on. (gay white male)

Devon regretted having adjusted to this shorter time range by giving up his education as he was alive and well far longer than doctors had told him was possible.

I was really frustrated because when I found out, they told me . . . it's possible that you may be dead within 6 months to a year. And of course, like I said that was 6 years ago, and I have known I've been HIV/ARC for 8 years this year. Had I known back then-because I gave up, I finished 5 years of college and [could have been] eventually going to complete a Masters and Ph.D. in psychology. So what need is there? I am going to die anyway. So I just gave up all my hopes and things that I was doing. (gay black male)

Peter had a similar experience. He turned his life around very rapidly after diagnosis in anticipation of a quick decline. Later he realized that he had to start living again.

I decided I was going to quit my job that day. I decided I was going to sell my home. I decided we were going to move to the Detroit area so I could get a better physician rather than living in a small town on the west side of the state. . . . So everything changed. Within 6 hours of my diagnosis, my entire life changed. After . . . I started feeling like I had some control over the disease, I realized if somebody asked me, "If a cure came along, how I would feel?" my response would be, "I would be very angry because I had gone through such hell adjusting to this. Now people are going to tell me I have to learn how to live again." And then I realized that I did need to learn how to live again. First you accept the disease by accepting death and then you have to go through the entire mourning and grieving process all over again to accept the disease, to accept to live with it. (gay white male)

The most severe reaction to the shock of diagnosis is reflected in thoughts of suicide. Peter Marzuk et al. (1988) report a higher rate of suicide among people with AIDS than for others of the same age and gender. People may also be pushed in this direction by the experience of discrimination, the threat of social stigma, or concerns about imminent suffering. Five participants mentioned that they had thought about suicide in the period following diagnosis. Sheila said, "Basically I thought I was going to die right away. I wanted to kill myself." Daniel also thought he was going to die soon, even though he had been told he might live for a long time.

> [My doctor] said, "You can be HIV positive and never get sick. . . ." I sort of believed her. I didn't think it was a death sentence to me, [that] I was going to die in six months. But after I looked into it, then I started thinking, "Well, yeah, maybe I am going to die in six months to a year." That's when I started worrying, getting depressed, and thought of driving into a brick wall and killing myself. But I got over all that. (gay white male)

It was the loss of his plans that led Jim to thoughts of suicide.

> I didn't feel like I was going to die right there on the spot, but I was kind of thinking, "Wow, this . . . really cuts my life, this really cuts my plans. I will never become an attorney now. . . . " I was kind of thinking negatively about taking my own life. At the time I really wasn't much concerned whether I got sick or not, because I was just depressed. (bisexual black male)

One participant in this study did mention that he attempted suicide fairly soon after diagnosis. Bill moved in with his mother right after getting his test result, and experienced rejection from his family.

> After 2 weeks I told my mother and them what was wrong, and I stayed for one week with them, and they treated me like dirt and asked me to move out of their house, and said they didn't want anything to do with me. And I was the most disgusting, vile thing on the earth. And that night I took an overdose of Elavil, an antidepressant which I was on, from the hospital, because they said that will help me live over the rough time. I took an overdose. I said I don't want to live, because I had the impression also they were really negative. And I was also negative, saying I would die from this disease. (gay black male)

Once he recovered from this attempt, Bill moved away from his family and got his life going again.

Two people with backgrounds of substance abuse described their patterns of drug and alcohol use after diagnosis as near-suicidal behavior. Todd, a former social service worker in his thirties, started using again soon after his diagnosis.

> When I found out about this, about testing positive, I just . . . went over the deep end. . . . I had also been sober from 1981 up to that point and when this hit me. I went right back to drugs, right back to booze and

really had a real hard time up to November cause it just about led to
suicide in my case. (gay white male)

The idea that her life was about to end led Ninia to "shoot as much dope
as I could, because I wanted to live before I died."

> They came in and it was like something you see on a soap opera: the
> lights were turned down, they pulled the shades, and they came up to
> me with solemn faces and said you have AIDS. Nobody offered me pam-
> phlets—this is the hospital. So it was that time I said, "OK, I have just a
> short time to live so I am really going to party." Because in my mind it
> was associated with AIDS was like 2 weeks, 2 months at the most to live.
> I knew nothing about it. All I knew was AIDS was death. (heterosexual
> white female)

Rebuilding

The sense of loss and of the crumbling of a personal future varies among
study participants, often according to their social class. Middle-class
respondents often experience an acute sense of personal tragedy as they
measure a new truncated future threatened by illness against the bright
future they had envisioned for themselves. Men, in particular, tend to
have a great deal of their sense of personal worth wrapped up with their
job accomplishments and for young men embarking on new careers,
HIV seemed to dash implicit career paths and life trajectories. Those
with a tenuous foothold in the world of work, and especially those with
a history of drug use, tended to hold different conceptions about their
personal futures.

More often concerned with making ends meet on a day-to-day basis,
they had less reason to hold long-term plans or career expectations. It is
perhaps ironic that these study participants interpreted HIV more often
as an occasion for starting afresh, reorganizing their lives, and deriving
some good from a bad situation. Without a sense of "falling" from an elevated social status, HIV could be understood as a break from a painful or
unfortunate past. (This redemptionist approach is discussed further in
chapter 3). Mike was informed of his HIV status after being tested in
prison. He took HIV as a challenge to be overcome.

> I wanted to live. I didn't want to die in jail. I didn't want to die in jail,
> so I exercised. They told me to exercise, eat 3 times a day, make sure
> you eat all 3 meals, the main important meal is breakfast, because your
> body be broke down when you wake up in the morning, and you have

to build your body back up. Just keep my mind more so busy, and think about living at the time, not feeling so bad about the future, what the future might be, because the future might be all right for me too, because they might come out with a cure by that time, before I get too sick. (heterosexual black male)

Kent Sandstrom (1990:290–91) argues that people living with HIV may develop the idea of a "special mission" which provides them with "a sense of mastery and self-worth by giving their condition a more positive or redemptive meaning." The emphasis on turning one's life around represents one strategy for mobilizing resources which seemed to have particular resonance among those with minimal resources at hand. HIV infection made some people aware of resources they had never called on before. They found themselves handling situations they would not have thought themselves capable of managing. Lemuel surprised himself with his ability to manage HIV infection.

I hear people saying I couldn't handle that, so I was like everyone else, "Oh no I couldn't handle nothing like that." You think of, if a family member passed or something, you say, "Well I couldn't do it, I couldn't go through with it," but you do. You go through with it. I come to find out that I am not quite as thin skinned as I thought I was. (gay black male)

Of course, carrying through with these good intentions can be very difficult. Lemuel had a helpful doctor who gave him a great deal of information about living with HIV infection. He left the office with the best intentions of living healthily. He found it was harder than he thought it would be to live that way.

Now I don't know if he perceived this or not, and I was very dramatic, and I walked out of the office, and I was just thinking I will live the rest of my life in like a glass bubble. I would say two months later [I was] marching back up to the liquor store to get some more Bud. I drunk beer. And going into denial. (gay black male)

Setting Priorities

One of the most profound disruptions associated with HIV infection can be a sharp change in perception of the life cycle. Charmaz (1991:171, 221–56) found that a change in the sense of time was one of the major adjustments people made in response to chronic illness. A temporal reorientation may require an adjustment in life plans. This depends to some extent on social position. Class, gender, ethnicity and sexuality all have a significant impact on one's sense of life trajectory. Some may organize their lives around a career while others concentrate all their energies on daily survival. Some may focus on employment while others emphasize domestic life and the rearing of children. Nick felt that he had entered old age prematurely.

> I felt like I had retired, I mean I was approaching retirement age. And it didn't make any sense but that went over and over in my mind. I had become an older person. I had reached that last era of my life. (gay white male)

Bill was in medical school but discontinued his education, despite the encouragement of many around him. He lost the confidence required for a long-term perspective.

> I felt I was doomed. . . . I was going to go back to medical school, and finish up my MD degree, but now, I talked to doctors and different people and they say I should go ahead and do it, but I don't have the energy to do it any more. I don't have the drive, and part of the thing is . . . I read and say, "Why am I doing this?" I may not even be around next year. I may not even be around in two years. This stuff can get you just like that. (gay black male)

Roger, a former computer worker in his thirties, said that he and his lover were within sight of their goals when they were both diagnosed as HIV-positive. Since then, his lover died, their plans faded, and HIV has largely shaped his life.

> This is always in the back of my head, as far as how I'm going to do my life. I'm trying to get away from having it dominate everything, but there's kind of no way around it. . . . I would say in '86 we were looking at, within a couple years, with his business and the work that I was in, getting close to $100,000 a year, buying our home and doing things like that and it just all fell away. (gay white male)

Alex dropped plans to continue his education.

> I was planning on going back to school, and get my major in psychology. I said, "Well there ain't no sense in doing that now." (bisexual black male)

The sense of a shorter time span leads some people to abandon plans, while others intensify their efforts to achieve goals. Duane, a businessman in his thirties, felt a real pressure to get things done.

Whereas before, "I won't get to Europe until I am 75." Now you have
3 to 5 years, you're going to do it. That is how your perspective
changes, because you realize, unless there is some kind of miracle . . .
that is all you have. Even though you may live 20 years you still put
yourself in that perspective. It is tremendous self-denial, an emotional
strain put on the person. I still get up in the morning and sometimes
say, "I can't handle AIDS. I'm going golfing today." (gay white male)

A similar process took place with some people who saw parenting as the
focus of their plans. Andrea described an acceleration in her activities to
try to leave her son some security.

So now I am in a rush to do everything. I was always the type of person that planned for the future, had certain plans, had certain goals,
and now it is like everything is being pushed up and I am just like in
a rush to try to do everything now. Now, I have always planned to provide for my son. But now it is like I have to hurry up, now I have to get
a job, because I quit my job to go to school. So now I am finishing my
school and that is my second priority, whereas at first it was my first
priority because I quit my job when I was working 8 hours. But now it
is like. . . . I have to save and provide for my son for when I am not
here. (heterosexual black female)

Her plans focused on raising her son. The uncertain future associated
with an HIV diagnosis had an impact on those plans.

I think the worse part for me is the fact that you never plan to bury
your kids, but now I wonder at what age is it that I will be gone when
he is here. I always plan to have grandkids, not just die before my son
reached his growed up years, before he reached 21 years old. Now I
wonder if I am going to be around for that. So I think the hardest part
of it is my child. (heterosexual black female)

Lemuel recovered the ability to make plans with help from a support
group facilitator.

I remember at the afternoon [support group] meetings here, the facilitator . . . had structured . . . a series of lectures. One was to set goals,
little goals, small goals, bigger goals. And I started doing that. And
then it dawned on me, until I was setting more and more goals. And
then it was like, "Hey, I got time." I had all my teeth done. I went to the
dentist and had my mouth evaluated. . . . This is a long drawed out procedure, and that is it, I do have time. At first I didn't think that way.
(gay black male)

Some people develop plans specifically in response to HIV infection. David, a secretary in his forties, and his partner decided when they were asymptomatic to change their lives in preparation for future needs.

> We did think that [while] we were in good health and still could qualify for a mortgage . . . that we should make some preparation and have a house that would accommodate our medical needs when that time came. So we sold the house in Detroit and moved out there. That was kind of traumatic. We liked the house . . . but we didn't really care for the area at all. . . . As soon as [my lover] died I put it up for sale and moved back in, because my family and our friends were all here. (gay white male)

A change in time sense can lead to new developments in spontaneity as well as new plans. Ron reported that his plans were basically intact, though he emphasized spontaneity more than he had previously.

> My behavior changed that way and . . . I find myself doing different things, like doing things more spontaneously. As for weekend trips or stuff like this, get it in now, start enjoying your life, do what is important. . . . Other than that, my long-range goals, I've got a good job. Sooner or later, I want to have a house and a yard and a lover and try to live the gay American dream. And I haven't deviated from that. Just being a little more spontaneous, the idea is if not now then maybe not later either. (gay white male)

Conclusion

Though AIDS service organizations and the medical literature tend to treat testing for HIV as a deliberate and rational process where individuals receive counselling before the test, and medical and social support following it, the experience of getting tested is much more variable. While the best informed take this ideal-typical route, many others—usually less educated, lower income, and minority people, as well as those who resist confirming a diagnosis they suspect is all too likely—are tested in institutional settings where HIV testing is done regardless of the wishes of the individual or in a manner which constricts his or her awareness or ability to give informed consent. Being told that one is HIV-positive can rarely be experienced easily or calmly. The advice offered at that moment can scarcely be fully heard or considered as a person sorts through the enormous ramifications of having to face a life-threatening illness. Yet that moment marks the starting point in a lengthy process of reconstructing a life on a new footing. With few ready-made social scripts or role models to follow, many newly diagnosed people launch into a journey of (sometimes painful) discovery. Much of that journey happens with the (eventual) assistance of friends, family, AIDS service workers, physicians, and support groups, although approaching each of these kinds of people can itself be an uncertain and difficult undertaking. It is toward these issues that we turn in the following chapters.

Chapter Two

MANAGING SYMPTOMS

The ailments associated with HIV intrude upon everyday life in ways that need interpretation and management. Such symptoms as chronic forgetfulness, diarrhea, fatigue, or visible lesions require interpretation by both the people experiencing them and by those who observe them. Both engage in a process of reading physical signs to determine whether they are instances of "normal" problems experienced by everyone from time to time or whether they point to something more serious. This is very often a social negotiation fraught with conflicted messages (Strauss 1975:7, 50–60). Caregivers may rush to judgment, concluding that a cough is a sure sign of impending pneumonia, despite assurances by the person with HIV that it is nothing special. Conversely, other people may discount claims about the seriousness of pain, for example, as nothing more than instances of age or a personal failing. This interpersonal construction of the meaning of symptoms involves an elaborate exchange where the symptom holder is called to account. Accounts can sometimes be provided for questions from naive audiences, who need not know about an HIV diagnosis, which deflect them down benign paths of "reasonable" explanations of the symptom. Accounting for symptoms can be particularly difficult when the audience is an employer (more on this in chapter 6).

Friends, lovers, and family members may be enlisted into symptom management whether this requires compensating for an unanticipated disability or helping to provide accounts (see Charmaz 1991:69). The individual burden of dealing with the physical and social consequences of symptoms can be partially alleviated with the assistance of institutional sources of support, such as AIDS service organizations, helping professionals, and peer advice. Support groups, at their best, work to build a culture of coping where problems and success stories can be shared. A few people take a further step toward collective action in order to challenge entrenched cultural meanings which make living with HIV so much more difficult than it needs to be (see Adam 1996).

Defining Symptoms

One way of coping with the difficulties around symptoms is simply to conceal as much as possible in order to preserve the greatest possible sense of normal everyday reality (Charmaz 1991:68; Weitz 1990:33; Weitz 1991:129). Chad, a waiter in his thirties, preferred to avoid discussing symptoms where possible:

> I have a problem being a 100 percent honest with how I feel, only for the reason that I don't think that it is anybody's concern. . . . If it is something that I know I can carry through, I don't think that I need to burden people with it. . . . (gay white male)

The use of other medical conditions to cover for those that might be associated with HIV is common (Sandstrom 1990:284). Ted, a school teacher in his thirties, explained his need for tests to his family in terms of other medical problems.

> With my family, I went through a lymph node biopsy . . . but I covered it with something. I would talk about the number of blood tests I had; I would cover that with something else. (gay white male)

Matt, a maintenance worker in his twenties, used common complaints about blood pressure and anemia to cover for HIV-related ailments.

> When I had the pneumonia in October, I had the bone marrow suppression, and so I just tell everybody, "It's low blood pressure," or "I'm anemic, that is the problem." People that I work with too. (gay white male)

Symptoms which do not disrupt normal interaction can be kept away from concerned others. Tony, a gas company worker, took this policy:

I try not to dwell on it, minor symptoms, with the family or close friends. I generally don't mention it to them. (gay white male)

Wally, a cook in his twenties, took time to assess the gravity of his symptoms for himself before letting his mother know.

I find it difficult because I know she gets upset every time I have some . . . so I am kind of shaky to let her know the symptoms that are happening right away, 'til I find out if they are serious or not. So I kind of play a game of hiding stuff, so that she won't get overly uptight about it, because if I have a fever she is like, "God, you are going to die." (gay white male)

Deciding to discuss symptoms may involve weighing the distress that such a revelation could bring to others against the assistance they could provide, were they to be told. Terry, a building supervisor in his thirties, described the ambivalence he felt about discussing his symptoms.

I know my friends. When I tell them I'm not feeling good—I'm really sick, I know they are feeling [panic] too. I am sorry I told the people I told, because of that. . . . Yet I am glad because if I need to talk about it I can call them up and . . . they will sit there and listen. (gay white male)

Disclosing one's HIV status always raises the risk that familiar routines and relationships will be permanently broken even when other people try to be as "good" about it as they know how. Several people with HIV encountered other people who were not ill-intentioned, yet persisted in their focus on health. They came to feel reduced to their HIV status, as others focused on symptoms (real or imagined), thereby displacing regular interaction. Todd described the furtive approaches of people inquiring after his health.

I've never had anybody be cruel to me, you know, but I have noticed . . . a lot of people that have a fear of talking about it. . . . A lot of them will . . . walk up to me and they'll look both ways and they'll say, "How are you feeling?" and I'll say, "Really good," and [they'll ask], "Really?" and I'll say, "Yeah." (gay white male)

Others sometimes make choices for people living with HIV based on anticipated health problems. Sheila was hurt when friends who had frequently asked her to baby-sit did not ask her on a particular weekend as they thought she was not up to it.

So that bugs me, that people put limits on me. Or if my mother constantly pampers me, "Oh are you tired, do you want to sit down?" It is like, "If I am, I will tell you. Quit asking me. That bothers me." (heterosexual white female)

Bob was one of a number of participants who mentioned that they do not like being treated as invalids.

It's like when you tell people that you know it takes you a little bit longer to do something because of fatigue, then they almost sort of treat you like a grandmother. (gay white male)

Carl, a hairdresser in his twenties, was physically active and yet found people treated him as if he were infirm.

I feel fine. I'm working out, I'm lifting weights. I'm very capable of doing a lot and I find it very degrading when people say, "No no no no you should go sit down and relax." I think that's real degrading and embarrassing. (gay white male)

HIV can easily become a master status, engulfing other considerations in the minds of friends or family. David could not simply be tired without others seeing it as HIV-related fatigue.

If you go in and you are tired . . . they look at you and you know that they are thinking, "Do you look that way because you are getting sick, or is it because you are tired?" And you just want to scream at people, "I am tired, I work three jobs, I didn't sleep all week, I am tired today, and I am not sick. I am tired." (gay white male)

Once people start seeing every health problem as a manifestation of HIV-infection, they are inclined to see even minor ailments as major issues. Matt said, "People who know I am positive, they have a tendency to overestimate the seriousness." This overestimation can even override the person's own explanation for a condition. Ron understood a cough as the result of damage done by swallowing the wrong way, while a friend saw it as a symptom of pneumonia.

I have other friends that overreacted, looking at me like I was about to drop dead. . . . I can remember one night on the way home from work, I swallowed and breathed at the same time, so it went down the wrong tube. And I coughed and I coughed and I coughed, and it did a little something, so it took a little while for it to heal. . . . And I had one friend look at me like I was ready to die; I had pneumonia; I would be in the hospital tomorrow. I said, "Get over yourself, I told you what happened." (gay white male)

Andy, a social worker in his thirties, saw this kind of overreaction as particularly problematic with people who were HIV-negative. They were all too ready to sanctify him, even as he wanted to carry on with his worldly existence.

> Or else you have the slightest symptom and some people with good intentions, usually HIV negative, will be putting up the shrine behind you and adjusting the lights—oh, you're so noble and so courageous. No, I'm not. I'm just living my life. Not noble, don't build the shrine yet. (gay white male)

Peter suggested that there was a definite pattern to responses he received from others.

> I think everybody else outside of the syndrome overestimates and everybody inside the syndrome underestimates. . . . Everybody in the syndrome says, "Well sure that's going on but that's just a fact of life." Everybody out of the syndrome goes, "Oh my God, he's having another problem." (gay white male)

The underestimation of health problems can also be irksome. Andy found people explained away some of his symptoms as products of aging.

> If people are not overdramatizing something, they're—"Oh, that's just getting old." . . . No, it's not just getting old. It's a symptom of HIV disease and you're discounting it. (gay white male)

Brad found that he was accused of malingering simply because he looked well and strong. His experience of pain was not taken seriously.

> They definitely discount them because of my size and coloration and all that. Even the people in group, "Oh he is such a phoney. . . ." And that aggravates me. . . . They're not in my body feeling this pain I am in. I live with it everyday. They make comments like, "Oh yeah, he comes in here with arm canes on and he just. . . ." And I get so frustrated. Why would I want to carry them damn arm canes, or a walker or a cane if I didn't need them? (gay white male)

The minimization of symptoms can shade over into an overall underestimation of the significance of HIV infection in someone's life. Roger was taken aback by a friend who accused him of "using" his HIV status.

> I have one [friend] . . . who can be a real snot about it. I had mentioned something about HIV disease and she writes me back saying she

feels I use that as a crutch. And, God, I don't think I've ever done that. (gay white male)

Advice may be irksome in much the same way as the dismissal or exaggeration of symptoms. Carl found it particularly irritating when people who consider themselves to be HIV-negative offered unsolicited advice.

Normally the people who think they are HIV negative feel that they know everything about it and they actually don't know a God damn thing about it. I just get out of the hospital and have someone saying, "You should be taking vitamins. You shouldn't be drinking coffee." Now I was in the hospital for a month, I drank coffee every day. My doctor said, "Normal." What are you telling me? It just frustrates me that people who think they are HIV negative think they just know everything, and half the time they don't even know if they're HIV negative. (gay white male)

Roger relies on HIV-positive friends for serious discussion of symptoms.

I probably have a handful of people that I talk to, and Andrew and Louis, my friends, they are both HIV positive and Andrew is still listed as ARC. He's not listed as full blown AIDS, and Louis is on AZT, but he hasn't had any symptoms or anything like that. They're actually the only people that understand the symptoms. (gay white male)

The minimization or exaggeration of symptoms by others can interact with one's own tendencies to interpret illnesses in particular ways. David became highly sensitized to any changes in his condition that might be connected to symptoms. He was not pleased when his doctor made light of a minor mark that he had thought might be a lesion.

And I made her [doctor] look at that, "Do you see that? It is there." And she was laughing and she said, "I would have never even noticed if you hadn't mentioned it." I very seriously told her that I see everything. (gay white male)

This increased awareness of health problems can shift into panic. Terry found it hard to distinguish the impact of aging from the symptoms of HIV-related illness. A small change could lead to serious anxiety.

It's very strange because it is very hard because . . . I'm 36 years old. I'm going to have aches and pains. I'm going to have problems. I'm not a spring chicken no more. And when things happen you always feel it's the beginning of the end and you are constantly panicking (gay white male)

Coping With Symptoms

Many of the symptoms connected to HIV disease or opportunistic infections can become issues in social relationships. They might lead to changes in behavior patterns or appearance. They might be visible markers of ill-health or strongly associated with HIV disease. People living with HIV therefore find themselves creating ways of managing the social aspects of these symptoms. One of the more difficult conditions associated with HIV disease in some people is the loss of memory. Kevin had difficulty remembering whether or not he had taken pills.

> My memory is not what it used to be and part of it is from the disease. Just, like two days ago I got up at 8 o'clock in the morning to take my medication. And I went to the kitchen, got the water and I came back to my bedroom. And I got back in the bed and I couldn't remember if I had taken the pills or not, so I had to count all the pills in the bottle to find out if I had actually taken it. (heterosexual black male)

The loss of everyday vocabulary can lead to serious self-doubts. The inability to perform routine tasks can seem to be a marker of larger debilitation. Bob said,

> We were writing out an inventory of stuff we have for insurance and everything and I was counting my belts and I had extra buckles. I stared at these buckles, trying to remember the word 'buckle' to write it down and I couldn't think of it for like a minute or two. Stupid simple words I can't remember. It really gets to me. (gay white male)

Memory loss can eat away at feelings of competence and control. Ted's lover helps him keep memory loss in proportion by discussing the pressures he is under and the other possible causes of forgetfulness.

> I really get frustrated. Sometimes I cry, because I get so angry about forgetting something. I just sort of break down, and say, "Oh my god, it's dementia." He [lover] says, "It may be depression . . . You've gone through a lot. Look at, stop and think for a minute what you have gone through in the last week." And that makes sense, and it works. It helps. (gay white male)

In contrast, Bob's partner chastised him for forgetting things.

> A lot of times I forget dates and times of things I'm supposed to do . . . or I'll leave something at home and the other half will just have a fit, calling me stupid and stuff. And I just want to haul off and hit him

because it's bad. Even I feel I'm losing it, I don't need to be called something over it. (gay white male)

People may create regimens, like writing things down or counting pills,
which help ease the problems associated with memory loss. Nevertheless
the loss of personal competences, taken for granted by almost any adult,
challenges the sense of control over one's life and even personal worth.
Others may help restore the sense of self or may increase the fear and
insecurity that memory loss creates.

Symptoms can unbalance routine interactions as both parties discern that "something is wrong." Irritability, for example, can be attributed to the "mood" of a partner, to a fault or slight committed by one
against another, or to illness. Physical symptoms are not always easily
disentangled from other possibilities. Clarence, a photo-journalist in
his forties, found that many of his ailments would create tensions with
his lover.

The symptoms, such as fevers, . . . create an edge where it isn't that you
have to take it out on someone but it's like here is something that may
not have been there. There is just an edge to my [lover], so it develops
an edge on me. His edge gets sharper, mine gets sharper, and there is
a crash. (gay aboriginal and white male)

Diarrhea poses more specific problems. Many people with HIV disease
find themselves facing diarrhea, stomach problems, or other digestive
ailments for varying periods. These are common conditions which
can often be explained away. At the same time, they can be associated
with considerable embarrassment. Spontaneity in planning outings
may be curtailed by the need to keep close enough to toilet facilities.
Roger described the changes associated with chronic diarrhea. "Yeah,
your situation does change. You got to make sure wherever you go,
there are rest rooms." There are also emotional issues which go along
with these practical concerns. Diarrhea can be embarrassing, both
because the toilet is so strongly surrounded by bounds of privacy
and because continence is such a strong marker of adult self-control
and competence. Todd does not talk about diarrhea with his family.
Roger was mortified when his mother began describing his problems
with diarrhea.

I was never so embarrassed. [My mother] and I did this panel with a
couple of other people. We were sitting up in front of this group of
religious people and mom said, "You know Roger has diarrhea all the
time." (Gay white male)

Weight loss is more widely associated with HIV disease especially among gay men. Lemuel felt his neighbors were concluding that he was HIV-positive on the basis of his weight loss.

> Like I had neighbors who would come over, "My you are losing weight, what is wrong with you?" People whispering, and you hear AIDS in the whisper. . . . In my case I used prior existing illnesses that I had, to try and explain what is happening. (gay black male)

Joe used ulcers to explain his recurrent stomach problems. Sheila found that people identified her weight loss with anorexia. She used stomach infection as a cover story for her weight loss.

> A lot of people thought I was anorexic, I had a hard time trying to tell them, "I am not anorexic. . . ." So I just told people I had this stomach infection. (heterosexual white female)

The use of cover stories becomes more difficult with 'visible' conditions that others might recognize as HIV-related. Kaposi's Sarcoma presents the double problem of lesions which may be in visible locations combined with a strong association with HIV disease. It was KS lesions that led to the dismissal of the central character in the film *Philadelphia*. Tom, a corporate lawyer in his fifties, found that KS lesions changed his activities and constrained his contact with others.

> So I don't go to the gym any more, because I don't want anyone to see me. Even if I were to go into a private room, and to see spots on my legs, which they might see, I am not willing to take that risk. . . . So [having] that available, like getting high on looking in the mirror seeing what I look like, is a huge loss to me, a huge sadness, and people that haven't had that also don't understand that. (gay white male)

KS acted as physical stigmata, robbing him of a sense of confidence in his own attractiveness and thus of the promise of intimacy.

> I stopped going out to the bars, I can't go to the bar. I can't be in seduction, meaning I can't find someone to touch me and hold me, and I don't mean in just a sexual sense. . . . and now that I have these spots I can't sit on a normal beach . . . without people being surprised about what the condition is, either making me feel awkward, or feeling uncomfortable themselves. (gay white male)

Despite his despair about future intimacy, Tom was not without someone who cared about him and found him attractive (discussed in chapter 5).

Tom and others, nevertheless, found practical solutions to the problem of the visibility of KS. Ray, a former maître d' in his twenties, wore make-up for social outings.

> It depends on where I am going. I don't have make up on [now], but if I am going out for dinner I find it helps. I'll tell you the hair loss bothers me more. (gay white male)

Richard has a cover story about being punched.

> I say, I was punched in the nose or something like that. . . . cause I don't quite understand it myself so it's very hard to explain it to somebody else. (gay white male)

For the most part, the norms of civility constrain people from asking directly intrusive questions about "obvious" physical problems, but Richard was once approached by someone asking about his lesions.

> Only one person has asked me so far and this just happened to me the other day. He noticed I had the KS on my nose and asked me if it bothered me to talk about it and I said, "No." (gay white male)

In quite a different way from KS, fatigue can indicate to others that something is wrong. Tony found others to be accepting when he changed plans because of fatigue, but also felt a real loss in his own capacities.

> Yea, the fatigue, as far as doing things, I have made plans many times and had to cancel because I am just too pooped. . . . [M]ost people now know that I am sick and stuff, and it is fine, it never bothered anybody but it bothers me when I can't go and do what I want to do, or make plans and then have to change them at the last minute. (gay white male)

People who do not want to disclose their HIV status in particular situations may resort to cover stories to explain their fatigue. Sheila's mother attributed her fatigue to another medical condition.

> My mother came up with this little story that I have Epstein Barr syndrome and you get tired with that. So that is what some of my family thinks. Then, anybody else, I will just tell them I was up early, going all day, I need a nap. (heterosexual white female)

Bill tells people he wants a little private time when he needs to rest.

> I say I'm not tired, I'm OK. And I just kind of pretend I am in my own world, and just want to be by myself. I say, "People need time by them-

selves. I just want to sit down." I don't tell them I am tired, I am drained. (gay black male)

Gordon told people that he was burnt out as he cut back on a high-intensity lifestyle. He eventually decided it was easier for him to tell people the real reason he could not maintain his previous pace.

> It was difficult, because I was sort of running very hard and then I decided because that wasn't a good lifestyle for me. . . . I started turning down things to do. . . . and people obviously wanted to know what is the rationale behind it. And for a while I just told them I was burnt out. I just traveled too much, I did too much speaking, put on too many things at one time. . . . Then later on I said, maybe they should know the truth. I didn't feel obligated to tell them, I just felt it would be a lot easier if they understood. (heterosexual white male)

Medications can also be a marker for others that someone has health problems. Some of the medication regimens associated with HIV can be highly intrusive, requiring a regular intake of pills spaced evenly through the day. Pills can be hidden to disguise the fact of taking medication. Mike made sure that his medication did not tip off his parents about his health problems.

> I got to take that medication wherever I am at. My mother and father, they don't know about it [HIV status]. When I goes to their house, I have my medication. I hides it. I don't know if they know what the pills is or not, or what. So I hides them. (heterosexual black male)

Taking pills in itself is not a highly irregular event. Wayne told people his pills were mints. Jeff offered other explanations for taking medications which pointed away from HIV infection.

> A lot of people from society take a lot of pills for a lot of things. . . . I've told people in the past who I didn't want to broach the whole issue with that they were anti-depressants. I told them they were a new form, experimental form of insulin because they were just those innocuous social situations that you get thrown into and they see you taking pills and they ask those silly questions and you, like, just don't want to say anything so you come up with the most creative lie that sounds reasonable. (gay white male)

Many people who are taking medications on a regular basis use a beeping timer as a reminder. The beeper may then require explanation. Wayne turns off his beeper when he will be around others. Jason was not too worried when his timer went off in public as he assumed people would not make specific associations with HIV.

> I have a beeper which goes off every six hours and as a matter of fact I thought I had it turned off and I was in the middle of *Cats* and right when everything was dead quiet, it went off. It doesn't bother me because I figure unless they're doing the same thing I am, they don't know what it is so I don't have any preconceived thing about it. (gay white male)

Carl worried about his beeper being associated with HIV infection only in gay settings. In primarily heterosexual situations, he counted on people not making associations with HIV.

> A normal person is not even going to know what an AZT capsule looks like, so it's pretty easy to get away with it. If you're in the middle of a restaurant, people do not know that this medicine—they could think it's heart medicine, or anything. A lot of people have beepers. We just notice it because we're HIV positive and a lot of people that we know are HIV positive and have the beepers. (gay white male)

He does not, however, like going without the regular reminder. Asked if the beeper was more revealing in a gay context, he remarked,

> Right, and in that point I don't use the beeper. I'll time myself and I'll keep the beeper at home. And then I use another container to keep the medicine, then I'll keep a closer eye. But then through forgetfulness, I like to be so that I'm reminded. So in context of hiding things it's pretty easy, in a heterosexual world.

Coping in Groups

Support groups serve a wide variety of purposes as sources of information, places for sharing experiences, short-term training sites, and starting points for long-term personal networks. While some people find them an important social outlet, others reject the social contact as trivial. The somewhat amorphous character of support groups means they have to sort out divergent needs and functions to meet the requirements of various participants. These conflicting demands were solved for the participants in this study by specialization, as groups served constituencies which varied by gender, race, sexual orientation, and drug use. Groups differed as well in their organizational objectives, ranging from open-ended, peer-facilitated gatherings to life-skill courses run by professionals for a fixed period.

Perhaps the fundamental function of the support group is to offer a place where "insiders" facing similar problems can pool their experiences in order to learn from each other. The transition from attempting to shoulder the burden of HIV disease as an individual to facing HIV in a group can be a liberating experience. Lemuel used almost lyrical language to characterize the change.

> After a couple of months of therapy I went to my first support group. And it was like coming out of a fog. . . . I started going to all of them, and I found [myself] coming out of that fog, and coming out of denial, and coming out of seclusion, just holding my face up towards the sun, and let the sunlight warm, feel the warmth of the sun. Just opening up, that is the best way I can put it.

Groups can provide a long-term emotional grounding. Dan emphasized the need for ongoing support to handle the various challenges created by HIV infection.

> It helped me realize that . . . the real need for the support group is that it is so ongoing, that you have to have something that you can go to consistently, because you are going to be dealing with so many similar problems for such a long time. (gay white male)

Support groups, at their best, provide a place to be candid without worrying about the sensitivities of family and friends. Out of the experience of facing a common set of problems and out of communicating individual troubles and small victories can come a sense of mutual support and community. People who have lived successfully with HIV for years can act like tribal elders to the uninitiated seeking a way through an uncertain world. Jason summed up what he got from his support group this way.

> I needed to know more than just personally about what AIDS was doing to me and how it affected other people, family members, and lovers and friends and by coming to the support groups and the training, you get the whole ball of wax. (gay white male)

People coming into the syndrome could learn a great deal from those who had been through much more. As Dan described it,

> I went to some support groups . . . and I found it helpful, just educational. People talking about going through different aspects of illnesses and things. What state they were at now. It just sort of reinforced, opened up my eyes how long these people go through things, and how well they do too. (gay white male)

Jim benefitted from hearing others describe ways they dealt with the syndrome.

> Once I went to the support groups, speaking to other people that experienced sickness and infections, it kind of made me a little more brave to accept if that is what is to come then, what I could do to prevent it, and what I couldn't prevent, just to deal with. (bisexual black male)

Groups could also provide medical information, especially concerning newly available drugs or doctors with special expertise. Lisa obtained information and referrals for her son from the facilitator of a caregivers' support group.

> [The facilitator] introduced me to the illness and to make me understand it. . . . and I carried a doctor's name and I gave it to [my son] . . . . So due to [the facilitator] I had got lots of information, and doctors' names on top of that. (heterosexual white female)

The experience of being among others sharing the same situation was one of the most important aspects of support-group participation. Jodi, a family member, described the importance of identification in these groups.

> Basically, there's just an understanding of the feelings without even having to mention anything. There's a lot of just understood support. There's nothing like saying, "yeah, I know how you feel." (heterosexual white female)

This identification was crucial to Nick, who participated in a group at Friends, an organization organized by and for people living with HIV and AIDS.

> Originally I approached Friends as a source of . . . identity that I am not alone out there, with other people. That other people are going through what I am going through, I am not unique. (gay white male)

Identification could also be important for caregivers. Barb spoke to a social worker about her need to talk to other women in who were spouses of HIV-positive men.

> It was her [social worker] that I told, "If I could just talk to one other person that was in this situation I would feel so much better. If I could just talk to one other woman who is going through this," and she said, "Well we could start a support group of spouses." She said, "Would you be willing to do that?" I said, "Yeah," so we founded a support group

and it is two years now. . . . That was the beginning of my recovery, my mental recovery. (heterosexual white and aboriginal female)

The sense of solidarity engendered by support groups flows from a sense of commonality free from the implicit or explicit judgmentalism of seronegative outsiders. Bill described this:

> People who are HIV positive like I am . . . treat each other like human beings, like we don't say, "Well I am going to pity you because you are sick." But one of us will say, "Can you go to the store and get me this?" or "Can you do this?" We treat each other like people. We don't sit down and get on the pity pot . . . because they are sick like I am, so they don't look at you as though you are sick. (gay black male)

Group Problems

It is not surprising, given the variety of expectations and the diversity of participants, that certain problems emerge with support groups. Support-group mutuality may result in generalizing misery as well as coping skills. Not surprisingly, groups also face various personal and interpersonal problems. Some group members may feel others are insensitive, boring, or too talkative. Groups may fail to develop sufficient cohesiveness to create the climate of trust necessary for participants to feel comfortable divulging sensitive issues. The organization of support groups can be a delicate balance between openness, to encourage participation, and structure to ensure that goals are met. Tony found the first group he attended was too unstructured.

> The first one I went to, a friend took me to, which was kind of open format. Most nights there was, I thought, way too many people in the room, and of course everybody just kind of chit chats, and doesn't—I don't know. I never felt very comfortable, and then there was a couple of times, a couple of people kind of jumped on me, "Why aren't you talking more?" I don't need this. So I quit that and I went to this one here which is just kind of a start support group. It is structured and educational as well as support. That I found very interesting. I like that a lot. (gay white male)

The sense of shared vision developed by many group members may emphasize the solitariness of others who feel excluded from the emerging group culture. Anastasia could not identify with the other members of a caregiver support group as her relations with her HIV-positive relatives had broken down.

> They were discussing their family problems. I got something out of it,
> but I didn't have much input into it, because there was so little contact
> between family, the in-laws [and me]. Communication had broken
> down. I was in tears for weeks. (heterosexual white female)

The ability of caregivers to participate in support groups may be affected
by their relatives' unwillingness to disclose their own condition. Judy felt
that her participation in a support group might expose her brother's
HIV status.

> No, actually I had thought about it, but he doesn't want me to, because
> he is not ready. . . . I know so many gay people, that if I went down there,
> they are going to wonder what the hell is Judy doing down there, and
> they are going to put two and two together. (heterosexual white female)

The question of disclosure and confidentiality loomed large when
Gordon participated in the foundation of a men's group for hemophiliacs. Many people simply did not want to be associated with an AIDS-
related activity.

> It had a rough start, because there are still a lot of people among the
> hemophilia community who are coming out of denial. They just don't
> want to believe they have this problem, or they were just afraid. They,
> because of their joint problems, are already stigmatized in their
> minds. And now this was the ultimate final stigma for them. And so
> they disassociate themselves from this whole process. (heterosexual
> white male)

While some people find groups with diverse membership both interesting and enlightening, others feel they have little in common with people
dealing with issues that do not confront them. Gordon's experience was
somewhat unusual. Before the foundation of a group for hemophiliac
men, he participated in groups then available.

> It is hard not to get involved with the other communities affected,
> because you see so many . . . And they bring some group of people who
> are just HIV positive together. It is interesting, because there is a whole
> cross section of people, and of course I have met other people from all
> different communities that have been impacted, and you can't really
> isolate yourself. (heterosexual white male)

On the other hand, Camillo, a white heterosexual man, rejected the first
support group he went to in favor of a group composed of black men
many of whom shared his background of heroin use.

They said, "You've got to go to support group. The only one I know about is Wellness." Says, "Why don't you go there?" I said, "I won't go there. I went there once. It was like 80 gays. I got the hell out of there." And she [case worker] looked around and finally found CHAG. (heterosexual white male)

Women Forming Groups

Support groups for women may face additional problems when compared to generally available AIDS groups. The women most afflicted with HIV and people with histories of drug use (very often overlapping categories) may have greater difficulty traveling to group locations, must often secure child care in order to get away, and cannot rely on pre-existing social networks for finding others in their situation. Andrea first went to a support group with her fiancé. She found, however, that there were certain things that she could express only at a women's support group.

We went to a group together . . . but at the same time we have to have our own individual groups by ourselves. That is why it is so important for me catch up with the ladies at the support group. Because I just wanted to be able to express exactly how I feel. (heterosexual black female)

Cathy was no longer attending a group at the time we spoke to her because she was concerned about traveling at night on public transit to get to a group.

When I feel like I should continue to go, I think I will go, but I haven't so far, and I don't have a car, and I don't like to go out far, and travel at night time. (heterosexual white female)

Domestic responsibilities can make support group attendance difficult for women. Paula said she was limited in what she could do outside of the home. She could make it to some activities, but there was a support group she could not make.

I never went there, because I have a lot of work to do at home. I got kids. I got to wash all that . . . I just can't. (heterosexual black female)

In one instance, the male partner of an HIV-positive mother went along to the hospital where her group met to take care of the children so that she could attend, but this proved more the exception than the rule.

Some women in Detroit found an innovative solution to these problems. They supplemented structured support groups with an informal telephone group. Paula acquired telephone service that allowed for conference calling and hooked women together from their homes.

> I get a lot of support, and if one of the girls is sick we all call on the phone, we got three way [conference calling] . . . There can be 10 people talking, all of us with HIV, so there is no problem. And other times we can't talk, because I might have company in my house and they know if I am not talking. (heterosexual black female)

An informal arrangement like this does not necessarily replace formal support groups but these women were also able to construct their own support system which fit better with the daily rhythm of their lives.

Mobilizing To Make a Difference

Out of the process by which people with a common concern come together to develop similar understandings of their situation, and thus an identification with each other, can emerge organizations with the potential to effect social change. It is this lengthy process of network formation, culture building, and shared discontent that has brought many other social movements into being. What is perhaps most remarkable about AIDS-related organizations is the relative speed with which they emerged in a context where disease-related groups have rarely taken a political turn. All the same, there are so many critical ingredients necessary for this kind of personal and collective transformation that only a few people ever become participants in such AIDS movement groups as ACT-UP or AIDS Action Now! (Trice 1988:657; Adam 1996). Of the people participating in this study, nine (15%) of the people with HIV said that they had become actively involved in AIDS organizations and four reported that their family, friends, or lovers had become involved.

For Jack, a caregiver, involvement in an AIDS organizations could only be a destination on a personal journey he had not yet reached. He undoubtedly speaks for many others in similar situations.

> I'm trying to get my head together, because it was in a fucked up place 14 months, even 12 months ago. I got to take care of myself before I can take care of anybody else, but that is coming. (gay white male)

In contrast, Bob got involved in an organization for people with AIDS precisely when he was feeling the lowest, as a way of pulling himself out of despair. He started with social activity and ended up in an executive position.

I had to get more involved or do something, drag myself out of the house and not feel sorry for myself. That's when I got involved, went to Boston. They had some social parties for [people living with HIV or AIDS] and everybody was together and a lot of people seemed normal or at least accepting. (gay white male)

For many, making a difference means volunteering to contribute to the work of an AIDS service organization. Volunteering can offer a tangible sense of accomplishment in facing the seemingly unstoppable onslaught of the epidemic; it can provide a means of bearing witness to the loss of loved ones (Kayal 1993). Jeff became involved after being helped at a distance by AIDS organizations when he lived in a remote location.

I just decided that they have done so much for me in helping me maintain a reasonable level of information and self-awareness and mental stability that when I got to a geographical location where I could get involved with a community-based organization, I would get involved in whatever capacity I could. (gay white and aboriginal male)

Peter found fulfillment out of his work as a phone line volunteer. It helped him recover from deep demoralization and isolation.

Oh yeah, after moving to Detroit, I sat here for 5 months in the house basically at the kitchen table. I didn't go anywheres. I didn't go to support groups because I was afraid to go to those places. I didn't even call the hotline because I didn't know what to say. . . . Finally I got hold of the hotline and became a volunteer before I could even go to a support meeting. . . . Between being a volunteer and attending the support groups, I think they saved my life. For one thing, working as a volunteer gave me a sense of purpose or a sense of worth. (gay white male)

Tim's involvement in AIDS-related organization both fulfilled a responsibility to the community and helped in dealing with a family member's illness.

I am on a committee here, that is involved with training volunteers, and planning various volunteer social events, and then I help cofacilitate one of the groups. I think that did it, being part of the gay community, and feeling it was a responsible thing to do. Personally my mother has Alzheimer's, and when she was diagnosed . . . one of the ways I dealt with that was to get involved with doing volunteer work for a hospice organization. (gay white male)

Tom found volunteering to be a way to keep informed in an field where
things change very quickly.

> Out of my relationship with the first friend that died, I found my way
> to Wellness Networks and became a volunteer there, when they were
> still a fledgling stage at Henry Ford Hospital. . . . That was the sneaky
> way of my getting the latest information. (gay white male)

Keith and Margie, the parents of a man with AIDS, became more involved
in an organization for family and friends of lesbians and gays after their
son tested HIV-positive.

> Yes, it goes back a while before this but this has bought it to the fore-
> front. We are political activists in various things but this. We have
> always done something. . . . Never tried to hide the fact we were par-
> ents of a gay son. We had our pictures in the *Chicago Tribune* [after
> marching in the Chicago gay pride]. (heterosexual white male)

Involvement in AIDS organizing seemed natural for Andy, who had a
long personal history of participation in the lesbian/gay movement. He
exemplifies the model of AIDS mobilization where the personal and collective odyssey of embracing gay identify and activism acted as a foundation for a parallel conceptualization of an identity as a person with AIDS
and as an AIDS activist.

> I had been very active and involved in the gay community all my life.
> Marches? I've been in all of them. First one we had in Chicago, 1970.
> First one we had in Detroit, fifteen years later. . . . It's just an extension
> of me. (gay white male)

Participation in AIDS service organizations also served as starting points
for greater activism for some. Speaking engagements sponsored by the
AIDS organization provided a practical apprenticeship in advocacy.
Devon remarked,

> Being the only black person in Detroit and possibly in quite a few
> other places who would publicly talk about it, I have been known to be
> in the van. From there it has just been one thing after another. (gay
> black male)

Conclusion

Dealing with the social consequences of illness can be a question of
accounting for physical difficulties in face-to-face situations. While symp-

tom management cannot be experienced as anything other than a personal trouble, it nevertheless runs up against much larger questions of the beliefs and expectations of the larger society regarding AIDS. Support groups offer a first step toward translating personal problems into public issues (to paraphrase C. Wright Mills) by creating places where people facing a similar range of problems can get together to develop repertoires of coping strategies, shared analyses, and ideas about how to resist both the physical and social consequences of HIV. They are, in short, creating a culture.

The differences among the many kinds of people afflicted with HIV disease mean that their circumstances and their solutions will result in disparate directions and "cultures." For people faced with meeting numerous immediate obstacles to survival, from securing food and shelter to providing for children, AIDS may not be their first priority or the foundation for political mobilization. (More on this in chapter 3). Support groups may, as well, rely on therapeutic approaches which stress personal solutions to the exclusion of collective action. The active stance of AIDS movement groups which stress community empowerment tends to be in tension with the more passive role of the client (often unwittingly) encouraged by AIDS service organizations. Only a handful of the participants in this study felt so secure that they had appeared in public forums or on television in order to help change the "face" of AIDS for naive audiences.

Chapter Three

DISCOURSE AND IDENTITY

Discontinuous AIDS discourses have emerged from diverse social networks and communities affected by the syndrome.[1] Black and white, male and female, heterosexual and homosexual, employed and unemployed people draw on sometimes incompatible ranges of personal and collective histories and languages in making sense of AIDS. These discursive disjunctures in the organization of experiences around AIDS are in turn taken up by social institutions, frequently transformed and recontextualized by them, and then purveyed back to new seropositives—who employ the reworked narratives in making sense of their own experiences with HIV disease. In this way, the subjectivity of AIDS, emerging in heterogenous, inchoate, and fragmented ways, becomes reorganized into systematic narratives that provide its subjects a location and orientation in the world (see Plummer 1995).

AIDS subjectivities have been organized around several competing discursive themes. Perhaps most publicly visible is the Person With AIDS (PWA) identity that rests, as Cindy Patton (1990:9) has pointed out, "on the 'coming out' experience of gay liberation . . . mobilized as a model for people with AIDS, who, it is believed, can create an identity and group unity by claiming the common experience of living with AIDS."

Here people label themselves, identify, build networks and solidarity, and fight back—a model that sets seropositivity apart, organizes an AIDS subject, and creates a social force capable of confronting established social and political institutions. Though this discourse and organizational model is founded solidly in gay and lesbian communities, there is no easy one-to-one connection from gay identity to PWA identity. There is no lack of seropositive gay men who avoid the PWA identity and yet, at the same time, this model has attracted some support from seropositive people traditionally marginal to or outside gay worlds.

This discursive system, as well, draws people together from a wide ambit encompassing those who, while seronegative themselves, are "living with AIDS" in their own ways, including many gay men who are "at risk" according to epidemiological criteria; friends, lovers, household and family members of people with HIV disease; lesbians; and some frontline medical and social service workers. At the same time, many HIV-positive people, including homosexually interested men, disavow gay identification (as the increasingly common phrase "men who have sex with men" implies) and feel little connection to the gay/PWA identity complex.

In contrast, for many women, blacks, latinos, and aboriginal people (always highly overlapping categories), PWA identity lacks an easy fit with experience. HIV disease may present itself as "another trouble" among people already struggling to survive unemployment, poverty, addiction, and poor medical services while attempting to provide for children and other dependents (see Farmer and Kleinman 1989:152; Patton 1990b:9). Melinda Cuthbert's (1992) work on San Francisco street youth reveals a similar pattern: AIDS may present itself as simply another risk among a number of imminent dangers ranging from violence to homelessness. The threat of AIDS as a possible outcome ten years away from the point of contraction of HIV infection, may seem relatively "theoretical" to people concerned with meeting immediate problems of food, shelter, and personal security. Organizing one's identity around AIDS as a first priority makes less sense in this context. For black men with homosexual experience, this orientation to AIDS is common, though gay discourse influences many. As a result, AIDS is often dealt with in Afro-American, Latino, and aboriginal communities as yet one more problem added to the crowded agenda of overburdened health and social service agencies. Specific AIDS projects similarly must respond with a multi-issue agenda because addressing AIDS means addressing other medical and social problems at the same time.

HIV-positive hemophiliacs have other strong disincentives against embracing PWA identity. Located at the opposite end of the public moral hierarchy from gay men and drug users, and having successfully won compensation for damages from a number of governments, they have more to lose through association with the other marginalized and subordinated people who make up the overall PWA population, than they have to gain. While there are some noteworthy individuals active in community-based AIDS groups, hemophilia is a category which has "worked" better than "PWA" in securing state resources and most hemophiliacs with HIV have avoided the PWA model.

Complicating all of this is the very powerful and pervasive discourse of therapy (Patton 1990b:10). Especially for people who have experienced drug rehabilitation, twelve step programs, or professional counselling, therapeutic language offers a complete conceptual universe in which to place AIDS. Therapeutic discourse is particularly salient in the lives of IV drug users, who are usually otherwise unorganized, but is also influential among many gay men who have encountered one of the many professional programs. As well, many people discover their serostatus as part of a therapeutic process, whether in substance-abuse counselling or another clinical setting. HIV enters this narrative track as part of the conversion experience from an addictive existence (which denies itself as addiction) to a new-found overcoming of addiction through (a dialectical) identification with it. In this system, HIV often plays a redemptive role as the impetus to people "getting their act together." Therapy psychologizes and de-politicizes AIDS, thereby producing quite another AIDS subjectivity that is much less susceptible to mobilization. Like AIDS activism, therapy offers an experience of empowerment, but it is an individual liberation that presents little challenge to outside institutions. The redemptive theme may also be expressed in explicitly theological terms for those influenced by religious rhetoric.

Finally, social class differentiates the ways in which people construct their biographies. Unlike those who find HIV to be "another trouble," AIDS enters into the lives of many professionals as the wrecking of upward mobility and the deflation of rising expectations. Yet cross-cutting these divergent perspectives run several common threads that draw together seropositive people of diverse backgrounds as is evident in the ways in which people of different backgrounds handle HIV-related problems in personal, family, and work relationships.

Setting Priorities

Participants in this study were not asked any "direct" questions about what AIDS "means" to them. The narratives which make up this section draw on reflections made in passing, when people sought to identify the underlying philosophies explaining their decisions. While the predominant discourse around AIDS might be termed "pragmatic" and secular, explicit remarks on the meaning of AIDS often weave together discursive strands drawn from folk theology, therapy, and other redemptive idea systems. Steven Schwartzberg's (1993:484–486) inventory of meanings[2], based on interviews with nineteen Boston gay men with HIV disease, has considerable resonance with the accounts given here. Schwartzberg found the following meaning themes:

1. "HIV as catalyst for personal growth"
2. "HIV as belonging": being "more connected" with lover or family; with gay community or humanity
3. "HIV as irreparable loss" of future, sexuality, and friends
4. "HIV as punishment"
5. "HIV as contamination of one's self"
6. "HIV as strategy . . . to receive attention, love, recognition, or validation"
7. "HIV as catalyst for spiritual growth"
8. "HIV as isolation" or disconnection
9. "HIV as confirmation of one's powerlessness"
10. "HIV as relief," for example, as an occasion for coming out.

A great many people reconsider their priorities given their new sense of the finitude of life (Sandstrom 1990:290). This process of resetting priorities may be bound to larger religious or therapeutic meaning systems. Marcel, the housemate of a gay man with AIDS, stated simply,

> Somehow I seem to look at life a little more precious than I used to. (white heterosexual man)

Arthur remarked,

> I started seeking quality of life, rather then quantity. I mean we all want to live forever, but everybody is going to go someday. . . . I have tuned into some of my own positives. I kind of found myself as a result of the virus. (black bisexual man)

Others talked of feeling some urgency in realizing some of their dreams. Duane remarked:

> I'm going to start planning 3 to 5 years. I'll see the world. Whereas before, I won't get to Europe until I am 75, now you have 3 to 5 years. You're going to do it. That is how your perspective changes because you realize, unless there is some kind of miracle, that is all you have.

Even though you may live 20 years you still put yourself in that perspective. (gay white male)

Another spoke of finishing the interior of his house. Evan, a caregiver to
a dying man, sought a change of career:

> I'm going to undertake theological education not necessarily with the
> intent of being ordained a minister but with the intent of changing my
> life in a couple of significant ways. I want to be more directly involved
> with people. . . . I don't want to deal at the level of abstraction that is
> required in a large . . . bureaucracy. . . . A thing that will be obviously
> needed . . . will be more people to deal with dying and more people
> specifically to deal with gay people. (gay white man)

Nick found that HIV had selected him for a "helpful mission":

> But you just can't fold up and die, because you are not going to, you
> are not going to, and when you wake up tomorrow, you have got to be
> willing to accept tomorrow, that is really what I have been able to do
> for other people—not let them lose sight of themselves. . . . We are all
> dying, everyone of us in this world, we are all dying of something, we
> just don't know what it might be. . . . We are the chosen ones, because
> we have been chosen to educate a few people out there, in something
> that crosses all walks of life, . . . a helpful mission for ourselves. . . . I
> feel like we are chosen. We have a special gift now. I hate it to some
> degree, but it is still there, and we have to use it. (gay white man)

In Martin Heidegger's (1962:311) language, the sign of the " authentic"
life is one lived as Being-toward-death, cognizant of finitude and organized self-reflectively. This sense of reflecting upon and asserting more
control over one's own life can take a great many forms. For some,
redemptionist themes, common to both religious and therapeutic discourses, offer frameworks for reconstructing subjectivity.

Therapy and Redemption

Thirty-three of the sixty HIV-positive participants in this study describe
themselves as nonpracticing or nonreligious, while many of the remaining seventeen Protestants and nine Roman Catholics consider their religious affiliation to be nominal at most. On the other hand, many
describe a personal or individual spirituality unconnected to institutional religion. While religious discourses are especially strong in those
who do go to church, religious dicta influence others, as well, in relation
to HIV. For many, religious accounts of AIDS are a source of pain, a

dilemma to be wrestled with, or a starting point for making sense of experience. For a few, who had found a supportive church community, religion offers a foundation for solace in the face of life-threatening illness.

Several decades of psychological research have described the widespread belief in a morally ordered universe as the "just world" hypothesis (Furnham and Procter 1989). When belief in a just world combines with homophobia, people with HIV disease end up being assigned "blame" for their illness (Connors and Heaven 1990; Anderson 1992; Schwalbe and Staples 1992; Glennon and Joseph 1993; Schellenberg, Keil and Bem 1995). Among HIV-positive people themselves, the search to place HIV into a just-world context can lead to some remarkably different conclusions. David, who characterized himself as "very definitely and without apology Christian," found that his belief in a moral universe provided him the comfort of anticipating reunion with his lover who had already died of AIDS. He said,

> it is kind of a peace-giving thing to think that there is an order to things, that there is a plan and a purpose, and that there is something more then just all the shitty things that happen to you. . . . I believe in something on the other side, to think that there would be someone there, and that Lenny was there, and that if I go there it will be crossing to the other side, that he would be there, and that is just very very comforting.

Others read HIV as a physical symptom of an invisible disorder that can be put right. This idea bears resemblance to the ideas of Louise Hayes, which have acquired a small but devoted following among people with AIDS, and with nativist theologies around Christian Science. Philip theorized as follows:

> I also believe that AIDS or HIV is just a symptom of something else that is wrong, and that comes from my metaphysical training, and people want to be fixed, they want to be taken care of . . . and they have to do that themselves. (gay man with Catholic upbringing)

Camillo located AIDS in a moral universe by pointing to its social consequence rather than its individual effect:

> I believe that God put that disease out here to bring people together and it's happening, it's really happening. (heterosexual man with Catholic upbringing)

Elizabeth asserted a Job-like belief in a just world along with some uncertainty about how to make that belief apply to HIV:

I honestly believe that God has some purpose for Rick going through what he is going through and for me going through what I'm going through and it's going to make both of us a better person and it's going to make our life together better. I honestly believe that. (spouse of man with AIDS)

Redemptionist themes were common (Weitz 1991:71). Among the participants in this study, these themes tended to be expressed in class-linked ways. People living on low incomes (who were more often Afro-American and had used drugs) relied on salvationist language to account for HIV, while middle class people more often spoke in the more secular language preferred in therapy. Ninia, whose son was also HIV-positive, read HIV as a signal to correct individual failures or problems. She felt that HIV communicated this message:

Like wake up girl, a beautiful miracle baby here. He was born addicted to methadone. He was premature. I think God has been wanting me to slow down for a long time. He has been wanting me to quit running the streets and using drugs, so he gave me this disease. He said, "OK, I am not going to kill you. I am just going to give it to you, so it will wake you up." And that didn't do it and he said, "OK, I am going to give you something to really care for and I am going to show you if you take care of the two of you"—and I think God kind of did this to me to make me straighten up, I really do—it is like, "OK now you have got it, it is in your hands. You can either blow it, or you can straighten up and fly right." . . . If this was a deserving disease, I did everything there was to deserve it, but not my baby. I went through a thing with God for that, I really did. So this was the only reason I could come up with. Why did he do this to my baby? (woman of Italian Catholic background)

Crystal shared many of these sentiments:

I don't wish it on no one, but I am kind of glad . . . because it brought me to my senses in a whole lot of ways. It made me really appreciate me, appreciate life, whereas at one time you know, I wouldn't appreciate me, life, or nothing else. I just didn't give a damn. This is a hell of a thank you for someone to smash you in the face with "You got AIDS; you are going to die," especially with him [son]. I can deal with me being AIDS, HIV, but him, he don't deserve that. (black woman)

People raised in Baptist traditions often make sense of HIV in theological terms. Marcia described HIV in explicitly redemptive terms:

I was still smoking that cocaine, even after I had found out that I was HIV infected. [Then] I turned my life over to the Lord. I am a born again Christian, so that helped me with it a lot. . . . I got a grip and hold of myself, and I didn't want to continue living like I was living. I wanted to do something better, so I said, "the little time I have left, I am going to make something out of my life," and I went back to school. . . . To me I look at it like a blessing in disguise, because it has turned my life around tremendously. It is bad to say that some type of illness and disease [had] to turn me around but I guess it was the only way I could see the light. Now I can see the light, I can see all the mistakes that I have made in the past. (black woman)

Bill found that recovery from an illness strengthened his faith:

God who brought me out of blindness and helped me, and brought me from the dementia precox, and that men down on earth can't explain it—so why should I turn away from God, and start listening to them now, when he has brought me this far? (gay black man influenced by Islam)

In the twelve step program of Alcoholics Anonymous the redemptionist themes of religion and therapy are often bound together. The therapeutic language of individual change may differ little from the folk theology of salvation. Those familiar with the black Baptist tradition and with drug rehabilitation programs often accounted for HIV in a vocabulary that drew on the two together; for others therapeutic language provided an alternative to religious coding of experience. Rhonda drew an explicit parallel between alcoholism and HIV disease:

It is somewhat the same, because [alcoholism] is also a disease. Alcohol is something that needs to be controlled. So it is all in that same group, and learning to accept you are an alcoholic and doing something about it, and learning that you are HIV and doing something about it. . . . I honestly believe that if it wasn't for my experience with AA, and my medical [knowledge] I would be a total basket case over this HIV. (white heterosexual woman)

Rick, who had considerable experience in drug rehabilitation programs, organized his experience of HIV along similar lines:

I believe there's a reason I'm at where I'm at right now and it's something bigger and greater than I am. . . . I'm not a religious person but I do believe there's a power greater than oneself. . . . I'm doing something very positive [AIDS education] and something where I feel good

about myself and a lot of times in my past I led a very selfish lifestyle
and right now I feel a lot of stuff, things I'm doing and that, is very
unselfish and it takes a lot of strength and inner courage that I would
never have had before. . . . That's definitely encouraging me physically
one way or another. . . . I get all these things, these obstacles in life.
They are opportunities for growth. (white heterosexual man)

Sexual Identity

Much of what follows was offered in response to the question, "Did testing positive affect your feelings about homosexuality?" This question was
posed to all respondents regardless of sexual orientation, initially in
order to discover the responses of people living with HIV to the widespread popular identification of AIDS with homosexuality. In fact,
seropositive men and women without homosexual experience in this
study almost never "blamed" homosexuality or homosexuals for the origin or transmission of AIDS. It proved for many, however, to be an occasion for extensive reflection on the meaning of "being gay."

Unlike studies of people who are already gay-identified, interviews
with people with HIV or AIDS provide an opportunity to encounter people with homosexual experience, without presupposing any connection
to gay identity or community. From these interviews emerge a wide
range of subjective locations and transitions in the flux of identity construction, with respondents "trying on" concepts of sexual identity, toy-
ing with and divesting them, assuming them as a bedrock, denying or
pushing them away, or filling in their contents in various ways. These
diverse responses allow glimpses into the processes by which people
combine discursive resources, experiences, and social interactions into
personal narratives and accounts of their (homo)sexuality. They offer
some insight into the issues of how men with homosexual experience
locate themselves within the heterosexist matrix of contemporary societies, at the same time as they are caught up in the most ideologically
charged epidemic of the century. For many, testing HIV-positive jolts
taken-for-granted assumptions and habits, becoming a catalyst for
(re)considering sexual identity and (re)juggling socially available discourse fragments for encoding sex, sexual orientation, family, and race.

Testing HIV-positive may reveal the contingent nature of sexual identity and expose the underpinnings of identity construction. To use phenomenological language, the test disrupts taken-for-granted reality, jars
the subject away from previously unproblematic accounts of experience,
and forces reflection and theorizing in order to assert a renewed sense
of order. That taken-for-granted sense of order is woven over time out of

a range of discursive threads provided by several sources. In North American societies, the primary culturally available source is a hetero-sexist logic which sets snares and tripwires for male-bonding men; the gay world provides an alternative cultural revaluation.

Several respondents offered testimonies of the experiences of tak-ing stock, doubting, and reassessing their sexuality in light of testing HIV-positive:

> At the early part, it did, because I said, "Well if you hadn't been gay, you wouldn't be in this position" and then as I have learned, as I teach other people, HIV is equal opportunity; he doesn't care what you are. I did at one time but now I am accepting it, being gay and being HIV. (black male, 35)

> I would say overall I am very comfortable [with my homosexuality]. I think a lot of it is doubts brought out by HIV and I realize where they are coming from, but they are still difficult to deal with at times. There is a lot of guilt that can be attached to that. (white male, 38)

For one man, these issues were mixed with issues of recovery from alcohol abuse:

> I had getting sober to deal with at the same time so it's hard to sort out which was which, but I had coming out issues all over again. I thought, this is insane. Why is this stuff popping up again? I've been out for twenty years. (white male, 39)

Testing HIV-positive may not so much challenge sexual identity, as raise parallel issues of disclosure. For many gay men, coming out had pro-vided a "first-run" experience of disclosing unwanted news to family and friends (see chapter 5). Remarked one man after the test,

> I feel like I was put back into another closet. (white male, 40)

Popular Essentialism

For many men, HIV did not challenge their sense of self, either because their sexual orientation was felt to be so fundamental a part of them-selves or because they had already developed a solid sense of identity beyond the dictates of heterosexist presumptions. For some, this took the form of a folk essentialism, pointing toward a personal origin myth or naturalism as the Archimedean point for their interpretive coordi-nates. Rather like the origin myths of the Plains Indian *berdache* (Williams 1986:ch. 1), one man simply asserts having never been anything else and being confirmed in this "knowledge" by "everybody" who was able to read signs of the sexuality which were always already there. From this vantage point, HIV is an external disturbance and no challenge to one's essential being. Rather, the reflective attitude stimulated by HIV status is about "getting it together." Lemuel opined:

> I knew, as soon as I found out what it [homosexuality] was—like before puberty. I knew what it was. But anyway, looking at it different, I don't look at it [HIV] like a punishment. I look at it more like, a get-your-act-together kind of thing. . . . So I looked at the virus, not that it is bad to be gay, but to don't take it for granted, get it together. . . . And I went through a rather flamboyant period in my youth, so everybody knew what time of day it was. (black male, 44)

The moral discourse built out of a bedrock confidence in "what is" allows one to turn the tables on the western traditions bent on giving homosexuals a bad conscience:

> As far back as I can remember, as far back as memory goes, I couldn't have told you as a very, very tiny child what it was that was different about me. . . . I always put that in the perspective of: That [dealing with my homosexuality] is your problem and you must learn to deal with that. It is not up to me to solve that problem for you, so you have to learn to deal with it. (white male, 43)

The essential gay identity is a discourse given out in gay folk culture, confirmed in the experience of a great many lesbians and gay men, and pursued by gay scientists from Ulrichs to LeVay. It allows for homosexuality to be a "discovery" of the pre-given, a fact so primary as to fully resist the onslaught of heterosexism, and a destiny that can be embraced with satisfaction:

> It was like when I found out I was gay at 19, it was like the light bulb went off and I felt relief, and I said I finally found my niche. It was great! (white male, 36)

Settled Identity

For the greatest number of men in this study, their homosexuality was understood as "being gay" whether or not it was supported with appeals to origin or essence. HIV was an entirely different matter. Scientific and medical discourses facilitated the separation of HIV from moral or sexual considerations. The cosmological freighting loaded onto AIDS could be stripped away in order to see it as something absurd, meaningless, or happenstance, not to be conflated with sex, love, or the gay world. To the question, "Did testing positive affect your feelings about homosexuality?" this man replies:

> No, actually I would say, no, it didn't affect it at all. No, it didn't make me feel bad. It happened. I guess I used unsafe precautions once and it happened to me and that is too bad now. But it's done and I am gay and I am happy. . . . I have told them [family] that if they want me to be in their life, then they are going to have to accept me being gay and that is all there is to it and they have learned to accept it now. (white male, 21)

There is a chorus of seconders to this motion for whom their being gay is just a "fact":

> No. . . . It's just me, it's just there and I'm not going to try to change myself. (Métis male, 29)

> Not really. . . . I wasn't going to let the disease make me negative about being gay. (white male, 26)

> No, I think most everybody knew I was gay by that time. I have been open for a long time. (white male, 33)

> It is not a point of hiding it; it is a point of not displaying it. What am I going to do, put a sign on the walk, "Look, I am homosexual, I am gay"? . . . I don't dress up in dresses, I don't wear makeup, so I don't have to explain it. (black male with two children, 43)

Being gay is, of course, more than a question of sex, but an opening to an alternative cultural vision of intimacy, domesticity, and personal fulfillment:

> Maybe there are people who don't know I am gay, but I am always me. If they don't know that I am gay because I am me, then they are pretty stupid. . . . I want a relationship and I want to live as normal a life as can be possible as a gay person and I want a house and I want a dog and I want to wake up in the morning and cook breakfast [for a lover]. (white male, 30)

HIV as a Catalyst in Identity Formation

The remaining men in this sample did not understand their homosexual interests as final or essential. Testing HIV-positive provoked them to reconsider their relationship to their sexuality, experienced not as sim-

ply "a part of them" but as "apart from them." For these men, HIV caught
them in the midst of making sense of their sexual feelings, trying out various modes of sexual being, and encoding their experiences sometimes
in conflicting ways. For some, HIV "decided" for them that they were
"gay," setting aside other options or self-conceptions. This experience
was lived through sometimes willingly, sometimes unwillingly, as a resolution of and relief from conflicts, or as a label or restriction, cutting off
some other preferred option. For those caught up in religious rhetoric,
HIV tapped a lengthy tradition of Judeo-Christian homophobia, result-
ing in painful dilemmas and turmoil.

For several men, testing HIV-positive had been an occasion for deciding "once and for all" that they were gay:

> I thought about that one right off the bat after I was tested and I real-
> ized that this was what I wanted to be, you know. This [HIV] is just an
> added feature, a souvenir kind of thing that you've picked up. (white
> male, 38)

> I think it made me feel a little more gay. I think it made me feel like I
> wasn't going to apologize for being gay any more. (white male,
> divorced, 41)

> No, I am homosexual. I did get confused about a week ago, but I
> popped out because I fell in love with somebody. . . . Everybody know
> I was gay anyway. (black male, 29)

As part of the personal re-assessment stimulated by seropositivity, some
men reset their priorities in relation to being gay in the world.
Procrastination, or acceding to social convention, comes to seem to be
less a contract with the future than a waste of precious time. Clarence
lost patience with the demands of remaining in the closet and decided
that his "discretion" concerning his living arrangements had short-
changed the relationship he valued most:

> We would go out to restaurants and . . . a lot of people would come
> and say, "Aren't you so and so?." . . . I would tend not to introduce
> Walter because of my position and my job. But that isn't important at
> all, and I think having HIV made me realize that that isn't important
> at all. Walter is important. Not only do I introduce him but I'm very
> proud of our relationship. We are the only couple that we know that
> has ever been together this long, . . . We love each other very much.
> (white male, 44)

For some, being gay signified not being heterosexual or bisexual. HIV was assigned the role in their moral dramas of blocking fantasies of "going straight."

> I thought, well this is it, if I wanted to get married and have kids, even if that were a remote possibility, it certainly doesn't exist now. (white male, 38)

These concerns could be complicated by anxieties about being involuntarily "outed" by HIV or by a sense of having unwillingly confirmed the heterosexist equation that "gay = AIDS."

> Sure, I would love to be straight right now, and married and have 2.3 children. I would, I really would. I mean I think I'm quite comfortable with my gayness and I do know what it is like to be a heterosexual. I have experienced that part of life. I think most gays always have, and some type of growing up, had a girlfriend. And, no, it hasn't hit the heterosexual world, so yes, it bothers me to be gay. First of all it bothered me to be gay because, before I even knew I was HIV positive, everybody assumed you had AIDS, because you're gay. . . . I came to support groups and noticed that there was a lot of HIV positive people from drug use. It was kind of a relief because I'm not as labeled as I thought I was. I really did feel that, yeah, I was homosexual. There was no getting around it, there was no denying it at that point. (white male, 25)

Folk Theology

Religion raises other problems in constructing sexual identity. Abetted by the media panic of the mid-1980s (Adam 1992a) which forwarded Jerry Falwell as an AIDS "expert" of the day, folk theology insists that calamities have a purpose and that homosexuality could be fingered for blame. While heterosexual people are never called upon to assess their sexual orientation in the light of AIDS, many homosexual men find they must deal with having their sexuality thrown into the just-world equation. For HIV-positive people reliant on religious interpretations of their lives or subject to the religious preoccupations of their families, HIV may provoke a crisis:

> It forced me to really look at the gay issues in my life. I have been living a double life. Even though my parents, my family, they knew, it wasn't talked about and I had to come out and say this [being HIV-positive] and that was real difficult for me, and I think HIV forced me to accept being gay finally. I had two choices: punish myself for being a

sinner and at that point to become Catholic or the other choice was to feel OK about me and that this wasn't a punishment from God. So I choose to be OK with who I am. (white male, 39)

I guess I have accepted being gay, which is new, because I didn't and I think HIV did have a big part of it. I was always what they call a 'closet' because . . . I was raised . . . in a very religiously orientated family. . . . I have come to the point now where I don't care what you think about me because I am not accountable to you, so if you don't like what I do, then it is your problem. (black male, 35)

Some chose creative solutions to theological dilemmas. Jack decided,

Yes I do believe in God, but I can't believe that he has put me down here to be a homosexual, to kill me so he can go, "Ha, ha, ha." I tried the straight world, I prayed to God to make me straight, and I believed and I'm still gay, and I still have homosexual tendencies, so if all these beliefs are true about God and everything and I really do believe it when I pass away, I got a lot of questions for him. (white male, 25)

Jeff reasoned,

I have accepted the fact that I'm gay, that my family has. I think I was having a problem when I was diagnosed of living honestly with it. . . . I wondered and asked myself, "Is this a punishment from God?" but I always got the answer, "No," but I did wonder about it, you know. (white male, 30s)

It made me think it [homosexuality] was the worst thing in the world. . . . I would go back and forth on this issue, because sometimes I say, "God." Then I thought about it. It's not the wrath of God, it's Satan that has brought this disease upon us. God doesn't want us to suffer and then if I am doing something, like if I like somebody, why should I not express that love that I care for somebody even though they are the same sex? . . . I am still straddling the fence kind of. . . . but more now, I say I am committed to the gay life, because of what I have. (black male, 32)

Religious language harkens back to the magical thinking of earlier eras with its promise of a totalistic cosmology where everything has its place and meaning. This logic allows for a coping strategy of petitioning the cosmos by offering some sacrifice in return for a favor (Adam 1978:ch. 4). Ron relates a breathtaking cascade of thoughts that led him ultimately to gay identity:

Between the first test and the second test, I was praying to God that I would come negative. If I came negative I swore that I would forsake the homosexuality and be asexual or heterosexual whatever I could do. I was totally over the gay experience, thinking that was my downfall. . . . After the second test came back, I said, "OK I am positive. Heterosexuality is out. No woman is going to want me or how do I explain it to them?" So I said, "That won't go. . . . You know you are gay since puberty, so you aren't going to change because of this" and then for a while, . . . I was just laying low not doing anything homosexual, not going to bars or going to any activities, and I just talked with my gay friends, and I have since got over that too. I am comfortable with myself. I am back to a happy homosexual. . . . My long-range goals: I've got a good job. Sooner or later, I want to have a house and a yard and a lover and try to live the gay American dream. (white male, 26)

"Gay" Means Community

While thinking of oneself as gay may always be an intensely personal event, it was mentioned by some as a social identity as well. "Coming out" necessarily implies "coming in" to the gay community; *identity* entails *identification* with others (Adam 1978: ch. 1). In considering the meaning of their homosexuality, several respondents referred to their connections with other men and with a larger community:

And I think it is easier [to be HIV+] in the gay community because there is so much likelihood that the other person is either going to be positive, or has been concerned about it, or isn't going to put me down for it, because it is like all-in-the-same-boat kind of a thing. (white male, 34)

Another felt indebted for the warmth and opportunities opened by the gay world:

I look back at my life and all the good things that have happened and most of it is from being gay. The friendliness and the friends, the camaraderie, and the family. I mean I found my outside family bigger than my inside family, my true blood family. Actually I wouldn't trade everything I've gone through for anything. When I look at how boring straight people's lives are and all the things I have done because I was gay and got "ins" to, situations, you know, fast life—no, I like the fast lifestyle. (white male, 31)

Another stated his indebtedness and connectedness simply:

I have to be proud that I am a homosexual and I want to give more to
the community that helped me be who I am. (white male, 33)

Rejection of Gay Identity

Perhaps most remarkable is the large number of respondents capable of
escaping or reworking the discourses purveyed by a homophobic society; a few, however, are swallowed up by them or make choices which
consign homosexuality to their past. Religious and familial rhetorics may
induce internal tension and a divided subjectivity. Philip remarked,

> I thought, yeah, this is probably a punishment from God for going back
> to a gay life or some thing. . . . It's my own fault and my attitude now is
> that it's certainly, it's some bad choices and mistakes I made. . . . I was
> very, very promiscuous and more or less, it was no wonder I had it.
> (white male, 30s)

Young, sexually inexperienced, and suffering from toxoplasmosis, this
man was living in an AIDS hospice after having been evicted by a punitive family:

> Yes, I wish I had nothing to do with it [homosexuality]. . . . until I said
> something to them [family], they never suspected. A lot of them don't
> understand why I chose to go that way. (black male, 21)

The following two men gave their sexual orientation as heterosexual. For
the first, HIV caught him "out," revealing his sexual practices before he
had made sense of them himself and forcing him to construct an account
of himself for a fiancée. Arthur was not unaware of gay discourse, finding himself at a loss to account for himself to gay friends as well as to heterosexual women. He recoiled at the identity politics demanded by clash-
ing gender and sexual discourses, preferring euphemistic pronouns to
the naming of his actions, and catching himself mid-sentence while seeing himself through his mother's gaze lest his language "betray" a dis-
coverable essence: "She knows I have always been—"

> It effected my feeling about homosexuality, because I had been bisex-
> ual before and, at that point, when I found out about being positive, it
> was like I don't even know why I did it. I had to think about the rea-
> sons. Maybe it was curiosity at the time . . . since that point I never
> wanted a relationship with a man, so I don't even know why I had a
> relationship. It has really changed my mind about homosexuality. I
> have got homosexual friends . . . [who] can't understand why I have

turned off completely to another man now. I told them, "Well, just let
me deal with this. This is something I am dealing with." It has just
really turned me off as far as with guys. . . . I kind of found myself as a
result of the virus. . . . I had to talk to my fiancée about that [having
had gay sex] and for me it was just real difficult to do, because you
might say I was in the closet or whatever. I couldn't come to terms with
telling a woman that I had been with a man. . . . I don't think my
mother was real shocked about it. She knows I have always been—got
along good with people anyway, so I don't think she was real shocked
about it. (black male, 20s)

The other heterosexually self-identified man had a lengthy history of sex
work and drug-taking. While in drug rehabilitation, he began a relationship with a woman and decided to shed any identification with the
gay world.

If it had come down to that [revealing homosexuality], I would have
said I was a drug addict because there is less stigma to it. . . . A homosexual is a person who has a very odd view of how sex relationships
should be and I didn't want to expose myself or I wouldn't have
wanted to expose myself to that embarrassment. I had let my family
know and at that time I was openly gay. I didn't think there was anything wrong with it, but if I had a choice—because when around the
same time that I did find out [being HIV+], my gay relationship came
to an end and I started to see women again and was more [into]
straight life again. (white male, 23)

Bisexuality as Anti-Identity

In an era when bisexuality is being formulated as a "third" term to be
added to the homosexual-heterosexual dichotomy, it is often lived out
much more ambiguously. Its interstitial status offers insight into how the
other two categories are constructed and a tool to help sort through the
tangle of family, kin, gender, and erotic referents that hold them
together. The use of the term 'homosexual' in legal-medical discourse,
from the late nineteenth century to the mid-twentieth century, mapped
out a terrain in opposition to family, domesticity, kinship, and love,
being assigned in contrast to sex, loneliness, and the anti-social. Much of
lesbian and gay history is about the development and assertion of connectedness, communication, community, sociality, and culture on the
site of homosexuality, a parallel if distinct recovery of new forms of family, domesticity, kinship, and love. "Gay" and "lesbian" have always been

about "more" than sex and indeed as gay/lesbian has been opposed to "homosexuality," so "heterosexuality" has had to be postulated in opposition to family.

Today, few members of European or North American cultures can remain oblivious to the richness and institutional completeness of gay and lesbian worlds; it becomes increasingly difficult to express homosexual interests without encountering, whether willingly or unwillingly, a realm of implications associated with them. Yet individuals may traverse these terrains in their particular ways. While these interviews show the relative ubiquity of homosexuality organized as gay identity and community, some "men who have had sex with men" miss or avoid the larger sense of gay sociality. Like the other constructs, 'bisexuality' is no unitary category, but may combine various elements in divergent ways (Paul 1984).

While a few adopt "bisexual" as a self-referential notion, others duck even this label. Whereas the preceding discussion included strong representation of both white and black men, the "bisexual" men in this study are black. In this, our findings are remarkably similar to Lynda Doll et al. (1992) who studied HIV-positive blood donors at ten U.S. sites in 1988 and 1989. Among the 215 men who reported sex with men, there were "no statistically significant differences in gender of sex partners among the three racial/ethnic groups [white, black, latino] during the year before donation," yet 54% of the white respondents identified themselves as homosexual compared to 34% of the blacks, 25% of the whites identified as bisexual compared to 44% of the blacks, and 18% of the whites as heterosexual compared to 23% of the blacks. They conclude, "Behaviorally bisexual white men were more likely to identify as homosexual, whereas black and Latino men were more likely to identify as bisexual and heterosexual, respectively" (Doll et al. 1991:28). While white men in this study who were previously married and who had children often identified themselves as gay, black men more often referred to themselves as bisexual.

Bisexuality as something of a "default," unelaborated category is revealed in the talk of two men. As John Peterson (1992:150) remarks, "These men may perceive their homosexual behaviors as merely acts of erotic pleasure motivated by circumstance and performed without affection or emotional investment" (see also Wright 1993:423). In response to the question, "Did testing positive affect your feelings about homosexuality?" Jordan observed:

> No, that has always been a struggle, that has always been a problem.
> Sex with men and women occur maybe within two days of each other,

maybe not even that much and I have always gone with both. With women it was more for the relationship aspect of it and with men it was more sex. I just look at everybody being human and everybody is fair game. . . . I guess I told certain people. They more or less assumed I was at least bi. In support groups, I guess they more or less want to assume I am gay. I haven't really talked about my sex life. . . . I have always been secretive with what I have done. . . . My family has always been somewhat like the Soviet Union before Gorbachev, more like Stalin. It is not something we have talked about, not even between boy, girl, the birds, and the bees. It is a taboo subject. (black male, 26)

For Alex, there is little language to talk about his sexuality. Married with children, he refers to sex with males as an action without involving questions of identity, relationship, or community:

I am a recovering alcoholic and drug addict. . . . I know I got HIV from homosexuality. I just shook my head one day and said . . . , "Just deal with it." It was something I did. Nobody forced me. . . . Since I left Detroit back in '79 it has been mostly males instead of females. I did. I did it. . . . I told all my family what the deal was [being HIV+], but nobody asked me how. Nobody. So I always said if anybody asked me how, I would just say I got it. I didn't go into the details how. . . . . Maybe they don't want to know; they don't ask. (black male, 41)

Lester's sexual experience had been influenced by his use of cocaine to "buy" sex from men and women:

Yeah, it affected my drug use, but not my sexuality. I was bisexual and I still am. I was picking up women off the street and being gay and that is how. . . . I got it, doing that. I have never had real strong relationships with that many people so I would go out and get a girl. I probably caught it from a girl. I really didn't deal with too many relationships. (black and aboriginal male, 20)

Joe thematizes the differences between the homosexual practices of black and white men, commenting on the fluidity of practice as opposed to the rigidity of categories:

I had had a lot of homosexual experiences and I have been and I am still homosexual socially and politically in a lot of areas, but I also live a heterosexual lifestyle, and at first I felt pigeon-holed a bit. No other person other than the HIV, homosexual person would want me. Well now I am involved in a heterosexual relationship and the person is negative. . . . I felt like I was a homosexual and I could not change and

. . . even before then I lived a bisexual lifestyle. . . . Homosexuality in
the black community is very interesting because it does not look like
homosexuality in San Francisco and so sometimes people assume a
person is straight when that is not the case, neither do they think that
or nobody in the community will. As an outsider looking in it will be
hard to decide for himself who's straight and gay. (black male, 25)

Norma, who gradually became aware of the homosexual interests of the
man she was dating, concurred about the ambiguity of sexual categories.

I don't know who did or did not know about the homosexuality part
of it. Other men have told me he looks awfully sweet. I guess men have
their own systems for judging this. He didn't seem effeminate to me.
Like the guy I am dating now says, "I have to tell you that he [former
boy friend] always seemed awfully sweet to me," so I don't know what
guys have been thinking. (black woman)

The "sweet guy" apparently expressed a warmth and openness to other
men which was not necessarily codified as a singular sexual orientation
or formalized as gay identity.

Heterosexuality and HIV

Testing HIV-positive carries profound implications for sexual relationships. As will be evident in the next two chapters, HIV raises numerous
problems around initiating and maintaining relationships, and around
family roles and support, for both heterosexual and homosexual people.
A disjuncture is evident, however, in the impacts of HIV on sexual identity. There is no equivalent discourse for "being gay" among heterosexual people whose sexuality rests safely in the realm of the taken-for-
granted. Like men or white people, who inhabit an unmarked category
which allows them to think of themselves as just "people," while women
and people of color are particularized by gender and race, heterosexuality can protect itself from scrutiny by a culturally constructed category
of the "natural." Heterosexuality is not subject to persistent challenges
and disruptions posed by an environing moral universe and thus lacks
the attendant theorizing which must cope with those challenges. The
problems raised by HIV for heterosexual people arise in fulfilling and living out the prescriptions associated with the roles of mother or husband,
but not as heterosexual per se.

It is only within a homophobic moral universe which assigns evil to
homosexuality that testing HIV-positive can raise the question of sexual

identity. None of the respondents in this study questioned why they were heterosexual as a result of testing HIV-positive. Some of this is because most of the heterosexual people in this study contracted HIV through intravenous drug use. Like gay men, drug users tend to see AIDS as a silent tragedy which befell a great many people before they could take steps to avoid it. Both groups are offered ready-made moral recipes assigning them personal responsibility for their illness.

For those who believe they acquired the virus heterosexually, the comparison is more revealing. It has been widely noted that public discourses about AIDS have depended upon the separation of people with HIV into "guilty" and "innocent" camps (Adam 1992a) and neither gay men nor drug users have had the luxury of socially assigned innocence. The hegemonic exculpation of heterosexuality deflects any inquiry into "heterosexual identity"—whatever that may be—mapping the moral universe of HIV onto a "guilty" infecting subject and an "innocent" infected object. The logic of heterosexism has no place for the kind of ruminations thrust upon homosexual men; in this system, one has been "wronged" while upholding the "good." Andrea felt,

> In all my years of growing up, I always did things to avoid things like. . . . I was never a promiscuous person as far as having sex. . . . I didn't do anything. The only thing that I did that did this was fall in love with a guy who was a user. So because of his past mistakes and his—I had to suffer in the same consequences and I get pissed off about it. I get pissed off with him. I get pissed off at life because I didn't ask for this. . . . A lot of times, I kind of resent him for giving it to me. It was his doing. I resent him for that. (black female, 30)

The same moral logic applies to the "guilty" party as Camillo acknowledges:

> This my wife right here [pointing to a photograph]. She dead. She died from this disease. I blame myself for it because I know I gave it to her sexually and I'm afraid to go to bed with anyone because I don't want that to happen again. . . . I went through a lot of therapy to get rid of the guilt on my conscience. (white male, 43)

Heterosexual relations open the way for a politics of guilt which typically maps the guilt-innocence opposition over the gender divide.[3] For women who have upheld gender expectations by refraining from "promiscuity" or other discreditable behavior (like hemophiliacs who are able to position themselves as victims of a negligent government), conventional moral codes give warrant for righteous indignation.

Neither men with homosexual experience nor people who have used intravenous drugs are accorded the luxury of innocence.

Conclusion

While one of the fundamental concerns of this book is to provide an opening for people with HIV or AIDS to articulate their experiences, there can be no appeal to experience as a "pure" or "final" touchstone of reality. Experience occurs in the midst of language and can neither be captured nor communicated without some social code or discourse that shapes it, or indeed formulates it. The voices reported here scarcely come out of a free field of meaning. People with HIV necessarily draw upon socially available discourses to organize, make sense of, and construct experiences around HIV. Conversations with interviewers can be part of the process of organizing meaning. As Elliott Mishler (1986:53–54) points out,

> a question may be more usefully thought of as part of a circular process through which its meaning and that of its answer are created in the discourse between interviewer and respondent as they try to make continuing sense of what they are saying to each other.

Linguistic encoding processes take part in a larger social environment of contending discourses thrust upon people by such powerful institutions as families, churches, media, medicine, and so on. Speaking about experience has an inevitably provisional and situational character. As Norman Denzin (1990:202–203) warns:

> A speaker is never fully present to himself or herself because his language never permits him to state with finality or clarity what he means; what he means is always part of something else. . . . The claim that a text documents a subject's presence through the use of excerpts from his or her verbal reports must always be challenged. An ethnographic text, like its cinematic counterpart, can only capture or represent that which is absent—the actual talking subject—through narrative illusion.

Part of our undertaking here entails witnessing and examining the discursive resources available for making sense of AIDS. Ernest Becker (1971) contends that much, if not all, meaning creation involves the fabrication of defenses against existential doubt, the postulation of meaning in the face of nothingness, and the protection of self against the terror of chaos. HIV at times works like a phenomenological experiment by rending the fabric of taken-for-granted reality to expose a seemingly unjust and senseless universe. Like hurricane survivors deprived of familiar signposts, people with HIV must re-induce a sense of order and stability into a fundamentally absurd event. It is a task often undertaken amidst an overdose of folk meanings about AIDS which need to be defused or dissembled in order to devise a workable reorientation to one's life. While some advice books and support groups talk glibly about overcoming "denial," some element of refusal may be an unavoidable and complicating part of the construction of meaning. As David remarks, in observing his seropositive lover,

> There is a real dynamic in if I verbalize it to you then I can't take it back, and I can't act today like there is nothing wrong with me, even though I feel OK, and you can't see anything wrong with me. If I tell you, I can't take it back, so John sort of operated on a I-don't-want-to-tell-anybody [basis] because today I might not want to face up to it. I may not want to deal with it today and if I tell you then I have to.

David's observation points out the situationality of the narrative coding of experience. Accounts change over time, and study participants often remarked about ways in which their understandings of experience had evolved. Our focus on critical anecdotes of social interaction helps show meaning construction in action, the stocks of knowledge and resources brought to bear in problem solving, and the social networks which help re-stabilize reality.

AIDS presents something of a naturally occurring historical experiment in the social construction of disease having come "out of nothing" in 1981. It entered into a ready-made cauldron of contending social forces struggling to assert primacy in defining the contemporary changes in family and intimate relations. People with HIV disease have had to piece together personal meanings for their encounters with life-threatening illness out of a wide range of incompatible and often punitive discourses. HIV thrusts numerous problems and choices upon people that must be sorted without the luxury of philosophical reflection; pragmatic solutions emerge in everyday moments. Out of the everyday practice of making a life in the context of HIV disease comes coping strategies which draw upon discursive strands rooted in family beliefs, religion, therapy, and "common sense." This is often not easily accomplished. Nevertheless gay people, black people, people who use drugs, poor people, and women—always interpenetrating categories—are constructing cultures of coping in the interstices.

Chapter Four

SEX AND LOVE

Having a serious disease can cause familiar presumptions about the course of one's life and future, to shatter into a set of puzzles that must be pieced together in new ways. The uncertainty and life-threatening potential of HIV disease can stress even the strongest of existing personal relationships and cast doubt on the possibility of new ones. While chronic diseases of various types impose many similar difficulties on intimate relationships, HIV strikes directly at sexual expression and may allow the seropositive person to be cast as a potential threat to his or her partner.

The initiation, continuation, or resumption of sexual relationships after testing HIV-positive involves a variety of issues. Among other things, those affected must work through fears of transmission, the complexities of negotiating safer sex, a social climate of stigma, and changes in sexual desire linked to health status. Many (re-)construct sex lives after testing positive through often tentative initiatives and day-to-day experimentation.

Certain patterns emerge in the process of constructing these sex lives, though these should not be seen as stages through which everyone passes. Those not in ongoing couple relationships are often celibate for a period after they have tested positive, during which time they sort out early quandaries. This period is often followed by one of looking for new relationships, during which time people weigh the relative advantages of HIV-positive and HIV-negative partners, work through issues of disclosure to actual or potential sex partners, and develop ways of dealing with safer sex. Those in ongoing couple relationships face some similar questions, as well as other problems specific to couples. Some issues vary between couples where both partners are HIV-infected (symmetric) and those which are not (asymmetric).

We thought that gay men would likely show substantially different styles of negotiating sexual and affectional relationships when compared to heterosexual women or men, yet strong parallel experiences emerged in all of the groups. Talk of friends, lovers, spouses, and fiancés shows an inventive diversity of relationships among these men and women with HIV disease, yet many of the dilemmas and the ways of working them out demonstrate a commonality of experience among people regardless of race, social class, or sexual orientation.

Single and HIV-Positive

For many of those not currently in couple relationships, testing HIV-positive initially brings about a withdrawal from—even revulsion about—having sex. The most common response to testing HIV-positive is to pull back in order to reorient oneself in a world now shorn of many familiar coordinates. With many expectations and aspirations acquired over the years now challenged by an apparently imminent life-threatening disease, many people take time to reassemble their projects and intentions. Sexuality is no exception. Several respondents chose celibacy during a period of personal reassessment. As Devon (now an AIDS educator) remarked,

> I did become celibate. I didn't have sex with anyone for two years. I just lost the desire. (black gay man)

Jeff agreed:

> You go through a period of withdrawal. You do. You don't want to have sex because this is what caused the whole problem and you just want to kind of let things ride for a little while. . . . [but] You can't be alone forever and you shouldn't be alone forever. (gay aboriginal and white male)

Similarly, Evan, the HIV-negative lover of a man with AIDS remarked:

I've felt diminished sexually. . . . The subject of sex has become so
freighted with significance and with hazard. (gay white male)

Testing positive is immediately complicated by the apprehension that
one's sex life may be irrevocably spoiled and that no one is going to want
to become sexually or emotionally engaged in a relationship of any dura-
tion. In the words of Camillo:

> It takes the romantic part of your life away. That part is over. You meet
> a woman. You go to a bar or wherever. You go to her place, your place,
> you're doing things, and you've got to tell her what you've got and that
> smashes everything. There is no answer. (heterosexual white male)

For some, the prospect of new sexual relationships is further overcast by
bereavement. New sexual engagement may carry with it a potential
sense of betrayal for someone who cared for and suffered with a partner
who subsequently died of AIDS. Widowhood as well poses problems to
survivors, with or without HIV, of "starting over" at an older age and submitting oneself to the perturbations of dating. For Roger,

> Elliot was my soul mate and I'm just waiting to see him on the other
> side. I'm not interested in getting involved in another relationship . . .
> because I would be looking for someone to be like Elliot. . . . If I never
> screw again, I'll be OK. I've done my share. (white gay man)

Meeting new people seems a daunting if not insurmountable problem
for those seeking new relationships. Philip recalled the dilemma this way:

> I wasn't involved at the time with anyone and I remember I figured
> that that was the end of the line for that. I wasn't going to have any
> more sexual relationships. I felt real dirty and unclean. No one would
> want me and who would want to get involved with someone who is
> going to be dead in six months? (white gay man)

Some wondered how anyone else could be expected to help shoulder
the burden of HIV, if only indirectly, by entering into a relationship with
them. The disbelief that anyone might be "convinced" to consent voluntarily to the implications of living with AIDS is sometimes complicated
by a sense of guilt around expecting another person to take them on.
Rick mused as follows:

> Starting new relationships? No one will ever love me again. . . . This was
> my favorite few lines and I used to whine about these and I really
> believed it too. . . . The chances are, you know, I'm not going to be
> around much longer, you know, so what's worth getting involved

there? And even if I did . . . the risk of possibly infecting the other person. They can never have a child. . . . And then the impact of, you know, what type of rejection or things that they would have to deal with because of what you're going through. . . . And then when do you tell them, you know? Do you . . . just meet somebody and . . . finally, it's time to go to bed and you say, "Oh, by the way, I have to tell you I have AIDS"? And that's not fair. Or do you tell people right after, "Hi, I find you really attractive. Would you like to dance? I have AIDS"? (white heterosexual man)

These quandaries appear, at least at first, to close off the possibility of future intimacy and do so for people often in their twenties and thirties who very often feel completely well. Among the many reassessments of future plans and aspirations can come a dread or resignation to the end of sexuality. Yet, as several of the above statements suggest, this first appraisal of the state of being HIV-positive may give way to an awareness of new possibilities. Through sometimes fortuitous events, this bleak understanding may be replaced with a sense that new relationships can happen.

Cruising/Dating

The prospect of beginning a new relationship with a seronegative partner seems, at first, afflicted with problems of disclosing and explaining HIV to people who may not be known well yet, and associated with a fear of transmitting HIV to a new person. As Kevin expressed the dilemma:

In the past, I might have been walking down the street or been some place and saw a woman and started talking to her, but I don't do that now because I would have to develop a relationship with her and then when I felt that maybe we should have sex I would have to tell her I had this disease and I can use a rubber to protect you but if it bust, you might contract it, and I will kill you. It stops me from like meeting new women basically. . . . I don't think anyone in their right mind would have a relationship with a person who is infected, not when you can have one with a person who is not infected. (heterosexual black man)

Frank, a psychologist in his thirties, concurs:

You go back and forth. There is a conflict. You want to do something but still you are afraid and you have a little bit of guilt. What if you give somebody something? Could you live with that guilt? (gay white man)

Jordan found the experience of dating an HIV-negative woman renewed his fears about transmission and continually reminded him of his own sero-status:

> I told her before we did anything and although we would get together from time to time, she always would jump at a little pimple on her face or maybe a rash that she can't explain. I don't blame her, but. . . . that has made me a little nervous about dating people who aren't HIV now. (bisexual black man)

For many, the acceptable alternative to celibacy was to meet other seropositive people. This approach ostensibly overcomes two major impediments to courtship: (1) the danger of infecting someone new and (2) the problem of revealing serostatus and thus facing rejection or incomprehension. Sheila hoped that an HIV-positive partner would allow her to pursue her wish to have children:

> I don't think it is fair to another person to have to go out with some-one like me, though people tell me that is wrong and I am depriving myself. . . . I always wanted to get married, have kids, and I figure I can't do that now unless I get somebody else who is positive. (hetero-sexual white woman)

One of the reasons many of the respondents in this study had attended support groups for people with HIV was to meet new people and estab-lish sexual relationships. Few, however, reported starting relationships of any consequence with another support group participant. In contrast, three respondents began new relationships in drug rehabilitation pro-grams or gay AA groups. In each one of these cases, the new relation-ships were with seronegative people.

The different experiences in starting new relationships with people in HIV-related, as opposed to drug and alcohol, support groups likely stem from divergent group dynamics. Several participants describe drug reha-bilitation programs as an intensive, structured, and lengthy process of reexamining and rebuilding their lives where they could divulge their HIV-status in a larger confessional context at the same time as other group members are revealing their vulnerabilities and developing trust with each other. The AIDS support groups, by contrast, tend to be less structured, more episodic, and have a changing membership.

The intent expressed by many respondents to establish new relation-ships with HIV-positive partners often does not work out in practice. Others reason that neither celibacy nor dating HIV-positive people is necessary, believing that a consistent policy of practicing safer sex fulfills the responsibility of guarding against transmission (see Siegel and Krauss 1991:22). Andrea remarks,

> My thing is I would practice safe sex anyway, so when I meet a guy, whether they know I have this or not, I am not going to tell them that I have it, but in the same token I'm going to have safe sex. (heterosexual black woman)

Safer sex protects not only a partner of unknown HIV-status but also limits the contraction of new infections by people who themselves have weakened immunity. Steve summed up the pragmatic approach as follows:

> If they would have asked me, I'm sure I would tell them. But I didn't feel that I [had] to put a neon sign out in front too. (gay white male)

Still, adopting safer sex is not necessarily easy or automatic. Devon, a gay black man remarked, "I don't care what nobody says, it's not going to feel the same"; Daniel said,

> I didn't like the idea of practicing safe sex at first but now I actually enjoy it more than I enjoy unsafe sex. Condoms, I think, are lots of fun. (gay white male)

Several respondents resented that the responsibility for safer sex often falls more heavily upon the HIV-positive partner. Richard protested:

> That's why I get so upset now because I've been hearing a lot about court cases where people are charging and as far as I'm concerned, these people are two consenting adults and the person who isn't HIV positive, he has just as much responsibility as the person who is positive. (gay white male)

For Joe, safer sex was relatively routine, though he had to take the initiative:

> If you initiate it, people are apt to think that he knows and he has reason for concern, and usually follow through in precopulation. (bisexual black man)

This responsibility sometimes extends to protecting partners willing to expose themselves to infection. A white gay man found that "sometimes, I mean I'll still tell a guy and he'll still want to do the same old things."

Telling New People

While not telling but playing safe suffices on some occasions, sexual relationships of any endurance inevitably raise again the question of disclosing seropositivity. But when? Some people learned inadvertently, or
through trial and error, what did not work. Crystal waited until a critical
moment to raise her sero-status:

> I tried, but maybe I did it wrong, cause I waited until he got in the bed.
> He had all his clothes off, he got up, got out of the bed—I am still in
> the bed. He was gone-you're[1] laughing—but that messed me up. (het-
> erosexual black woman)

Daniel delayed his disclosure for several weeks:

> With one guy I waited six weeks to tell and he got very upset. Maybe I
> thought, well, maybe I should just wait and tell him after he gets really
> close and falls in love with me, you know, and when I tell him, it will be
> too hard for him to reject me, but I don't think that was fair to him and
> I wouldn't do that to anybody again. . . . Since then I've dated about
> five guys and I've told each one immediately. I tell them on the first
> date. Every single one of them has said, "Thank you for telling me."
> (gay white male)

Nearly everyone expects the worst in revealing their HIV-positivity, but
many are pleasantly surprised. One gay man recalled that his first disclosure of sero-status to someone he met at a bar elicited the same disclosure by the other man. Other gay men shared the same experience.
A bisexual man found that the woman he was seeing at the time then
revealed a life-threatening disease to him that she had been concealing.
   Virtually every respondent with experience in disclosing their HIV-status to new people had positive stories to tell. After several weeks of agonizing over confessing to a woman he had dated but not had sex with,
Rick could scarcely believe her response:

> It didn't mean anything to her. It really didn't. And I thought, "This
> girl's sick. There's something wrong with her." . . . It's almost two
> years now. She's still here. She still supports me 100%. (heterosexual
> white male)

Jeff had a similar experience:

> I phoned up and said, "I want to start a relationship with you, but," I
> said, "to tell you the truth, I'm seropositive and we must know that
> upfront because I ain't going to pull any punches." He was very good

about taking it all in stride and said, "That's OK, I'm glad you told me."
. . . He thanked me. He said other people wouldn't be as forward, as brave, that kind of thing. We started a relationship. It lasted a year and a half—good, healthy fun, sexually fulfilling, socially fulfilling. (gay aboriginal and white male)

For those most experienced in the area, there was agreement that "sooner is better" made the best policy. While some preferred to disclose on the second date, others had become used to telling right at the beginning. Devon stated,

I tell them even before we hold hands because I don't want to waste my time falling in love with somebody and then find out, "No, I can't deal with that." (gay black man)

Andy summed up the reactions he had received from his disclosures this way:

Usually they're going to nominate me for sainthood and how courageous I am or a lot of times, they're very blasé and couldn't care less. Very rarely do I get much of a reaction. People seem to live with it OK. And the more you tell people, the easier it is. (white gay man)

From the viewpoint of the HIV-negative partner, entering a new relationship with a HIV-positive may come with some trepidation. Linda recounted:

I was very scared but I trusted him. Anything I wanted to know, he would tell me. . . . He was completely open from day one. It was a long time before we had sex. I think he gave me about 5,000 backrubs. (heterosexual white woman)

Of course, not everyone takes the news well. Bob recounted:

I was dating somebody for a short time. Then he called me up and said, "Well, my therapist said I shouldn't date you cause you're going to die soon." . . . I was just furious. (gay white male)

Another found that the woman he was dating seemed fine with his serostatus until he first became ill.

Several respondents found methods to ease the way to self-revelation. For some, discussion of AIDS work, affiliation with an AIDS organization, or participation in a support group provided a conversational stratagem for "feeling out" the other person's views on HIV. Others permitted themselves to be seen taking pills every four hours or carried a pill timer with them, both of which function in the gay community as an "early warning system" to "tip off" those around them. Devon checked out other people's views on AIDS first:

> I just bring up the subject. I say, "Well a lot of people are talking about HIV" just basically to get an idea, their reaction. They can explode. They get paranoid and don't want to talk about it. Well then I know they are not the person to discuss this with. (gay black man)

Finally, it must be noted that in several instances, disclosure of seropositivity has entirely unexpected results. While most people with HIV, especially soon after testing positive, worry about stigma and rejection, several respondents brought up occasions where they had intentionally revealed their HIV-status in order to put off unwanted suitors. Crystal reported this incident:

> I said, "Look, we can never, never be intimate. We could be friends, but we can never be intimate" and he was like, "Why?" I took a deep breath and I told him. . . . and he said, "Yeah OK, I hear what you are saying, so when can we get together?. . . . I read the papers. I know how to use condoms. They are all right with me." . . . He was the only one who left me speechless. (heterosexual black woman)

Similarly Jordan wielded his HIV status to cool off a relationship he intended to leave:

> Actually I was hoping that this would drive her off. . . . At first she was angry at me. . . . and I just thought that when I found out, this would be the final straw . . . and then she started calling me back . . . and then she started asking about getting back together again. (black bisexual male)

Frank complained:

> I was telling the person so that, actually, I wanted to put them off and it didn't put them off in the least. They just were very aggressive about it, so aggressive that it put me off. (white gay man)

The act of confession itself may have an erotic component to it. The revelation of a potentially discreditable aspect of self carries with it at least an implicit appeal for trust and compassion by the other. Indeed this exposure of the self may be read as an opening for a corresponding confession or expression of support as in the examples of others telling of their illnesses mentioned above. The Alcoholics Anonymous and drug rehabilitation groups function similarly to create mutually sup-

portive bonds among its members which, in certain instances, grow into
sexual relationships. One man was surprised to find that, more than
once, women approached him after he made public presentations as a
person with AIDS that followed a confessional mode developed in drug
rehabilitation therapy. One woman disclosed her sero-status to a former
boyfriend who replied, "if you ever get divorced from your husband,
you can come back." A call to a former lover to finalize a property settlement in a will resulted in the lover leaving a job in another city in
order to move back to resume the relationship with the man who called.
AIDS may come to function as a trope in a romantic discourse which
inserts the other as the hero now able to demonstrate his love to the
damsel in distress. Our respondents had no problem shifting the gender terms of this formula to become rescuing heroines or comrades to
fallen warriors.[2]

At least in certain circles, a subtext that confers a slightly transcen-
dental quality to people with AIDS, is discernible (Herek 1990), the supplementary obverse of the hegemonic text which has written people
with AIDS alternately as victims or demons. It is as if the cultural construction of people with AIDS jolts them out of the plane of the "ordi-
nary" toward both the "demonic" (Watney 1987; Adam 1992a) and the
"angelic," the converse category upon which the "demonic" depends.
This dual extraordinary status can be observed among other stigmatized
and oppressed peoples (Adam 1978:44).

Couples

In this study as in others, those in coupled relationships, for the most
part, express a "high degree of support from their lover and high degree
of satisfaction with that relationship" (Wolcott et al. 1986:399). As Peter
responded:

> After my diagnosis, . . . he's been there every single minute. . . . He's
> been very understanding. (gay white male)

HIV can be a potent reminder of mortality leading both partners to
reflect upon the value of their relationship and of the need not to take
it for granted (see Interrante 1987; Bérubé 1988; Murphy and Perry
1988; Pearlin, Semple and Turner 1988:508; Grimshaw 1989; Maj
1991:162; Weitz 1991:110). Robbie described it this way:

> It's drawn my lover and I together closer. We've had a very wonderful
> relationship the last six years, and, um, now it's . . . moved on to a bet-

ter level. . . . Initially, it starts off as sort of a sexual thing, and it's evolved into a sort of loving relationship where sex isn't the keynote thing. Because we don't know how much time we will have together, we're doing a lot of fun things together. . . . My other half used to take students to Europe each summer and I would stay home kind of thing. Well now he's not doing that and we're going together, so that's improved. . . . We sit down and have really great discussions and debates about stuff that I'm writing about or that he's doing.

Nevertheless, HIV brings with it a range of new problems, often charting disparate life courses for each partner whether both or only one is seropositive. Nick remarks:

I think initially it brought us closer together . . . but both of us at the time were symptom free. Neither one of us were sick, and as times changed, it doesn't distance us, but it separates us, because each one of us is going through a different set of circumstances in the same environment. . . . But there is a certain camaraderie, kindredship, close identity, relationship, that is able to survive. (gay white male)

As Mario Maj (1991:162) notes, AIDS caregiving imposes an array of responsibilities: "running the household, providing nursing care to the person with AIDS, managing finances and legal matters, participating in medical decisions and serving as a liaison between the person with AIDS and his or her social network." Sometimes people with HIV may even question why their partners go on with it (Weitz 1991:111). Clarence characterized the situation this way:

Sometimes it's too much, it's too much for Nigel who's the healthier of the two; he's had no AIDS-related conditions, just tested positive. For him it gets to be too much sometimes, having to deal with my illness and my medication and by the time I work eight hours and have a groschen . . . to hook up . . . there are times when I am passed out. (gay white and aboriginal male)

Talking/Not Talking

Striking a balance between talking too little and talking too much about HIV is not always easy. The spouse or lover of an HIV-positive person may not want to bring up the subject too much for fear of "reminding" the other person of AIDS too often, while the person with HIV disease may find the "tiptoe-ing" around the AIDS issue to be stifling when there are serious issues to be discussed. On the other hand, friends and housemates may become overconcerned about HIV disease, thinking that every cough is a sign of AIDS, while the person in the syndrome just wants to have a break from having to think about it everyday. Robbie said of his HIV-negative partner:

> My lover is really bent out of shape if we try to talk about it very much. He just gets very nervous and scared. (gay white male)

Frank agreed, saying:

> I would definitely like to talk about it more. . . . It would alleviate a lot of tension that I build up about certain things that happen to me in my daily life. (gay white male)

Ninia explained it this way:

> I am constantly protecting his feelings and I am always afraid I am going to hurt him. . . . I have so many fears. I am scared to lay these fears on him because I don't want him to be afraid. See, we protect each other . . . It is so unhealthy for us because we don't talk. (heterosexual white female)

Especially at the beginning, people often sort through conflicting emotions and changing expectations, feeling unable to put all these feeling into words. Peter summed up the first months after he tested HIV-positive this way:

> It was a very, very hard period for both of us. I mean he was accepting the fact that I was going to die and I was accepting the fact that I was going to die and we were just trying to work apart from each other. . . . After we got to the point that we both decided that I was going to continue to live with the disease, the intimacy went back to basically where today . . . [it is where] it used to be before the diagnosis. (gay white male)

When one or both of the partners in a current relationship test HIV-positive, couples often must actively adjust comfortable, routinized, and well-liked patterns of interaction. These adjustments may vary between symmetric (couples where both partners are HIV-positive) and asymmetric couples (where only one partner is seropositive). Despite a widespread perception of the abandonment of people with AIDS by their domestic partners propagated by the media in the mid-1980s (Altman 1986:60), HIV was no more than a minor factor in the few post-test breakups of couples reported here. On the contrary, in several instances, the partner with HIV initiated distancing or breakup after testing positive. Like the single people reviewed above, many partnered individuals experience a sense of desexualization, withdrawal, and worthlessness after diagnosis. Fred put it this way:

> I just started to push away. In other words, I wanted to end this relationship. I don't want to subject anyone to what is wrong with me and eventually it did end and it ended on a very good note, not a bad note. I keep in touch with his parents now; they keep in touch with me. (gay black man)

Ninia remarked of her husband:

> He hates condoms—and I would feel guilty about that because it would take him longer to climax. Oh God, this is all my fault; he wouldn't have to do this if it weren't for me. So we just quit having sex for quite a while. (heterosexual white female)

Caregivers sometimes experience a similar reluctance on the part of their domestic partners. After diagnosis, Doug found that his lover was "standoffish."

> Any move I was trying to make towards him was like, no, get away, get away from me, because he didn't want to hurt me . . . figuring we're going to get too deep into this and it's too scary for him. So I had to break though that barrier and when I did and started just mutual masturbation for sexual contact and what not, it was like somebody took a ton of weight off of his back. (gay white male)

Problems in the introduction of safer sex practices arise in both symmetric couples, who attend to warnings by public health officials of the danger of reinfection, and in asymmetric couples who must guard against HIV transmission. Barb expressed the problem of coping with the message implied by the introduction of condoms into relationships:

> The issue is we never used them before. . . . Because he has to use them now, what does that mean? That means that he could give me—that he is a vector of disease. That is, psychologically, it takes away from the fun part of it. . . . Unfortunately we have not gotten to the point where we could . . . resume where we had left off years ago. (heterosexual white and aboriginal female)

For gay male couples who had heard the safer sex message many times before, the adjustment is sometimes smoother. Wayne described changes in matter-of-fact terms.

We don't enter each other or fist. We learned new turn-ons—or to us anyway—putting a rubber on each other, that is a turn-on now. (gay white male)

Nearly all of the symmetric couples in this study stated firmly that the transition to safer sex had been made and remained a consistent policy in their relationships.

The adoption of safer sex proved difficult in several asymmetric couples and, again, in several instances, the seropositive person felt responsible for its introduction:

As far as sexual activity . . . I have to encourage her now and then or remind her what's safe, what's not safe and be careful. (white heterosexual male)

Sometimes he act like he can't wait and I might be sleepy but he does stuck me, but he still straight [HIV-negative] thank God. But he not worried about that. I be the one that be saying, "Use a condom." (black heterosexual female)

We had a real hard time dealing with that one because my lover really didn't see any purpose in safe sex and he said, "We've been doing it this way for six years and I haven't become positive yet. . . . I'm obviously not going to get it from you." (white gay male)

The seronegative partner may feel, however, that he or she is being kept to too strict a standard of safety. Ian complained:

Safer sex is not obnoxious but it's a restriction . . . . Everything that is listed as safe sex, mutual masturbation, . . . is not my cup of tea. Condom use is OK but he rejects the idea of doing anal intercourse with a condom because condoms are not 100% safe. (gay white male)

A "rational person" model of sexual behavior might predict that asymmetric couples would be quicker to adopt safer sex given the imperative to protect the uninfected partner, whereas failure to practice safer sex among symmetric couples might be more likely as it leads to less serious and more abstract consequences.

The examples here suggest a deeper logic and a different conclusion flowing out of a complex and treacherous interplay of meanings. The asymmetric test result violates a fundamental property of couples by rupturing their sense of a shared fate in its designation of one partner as marked by a life-threatening disease and as a potential threat to the other. In some sense, the HIV-negative partner may seek to abstain from confirming this script by refusing to comply with this stigmatization of his or her partner through failing to protect him- or herself from the imputed threat of infection.[3] While the shift toward safer sex among symmetric couples can remain consistent with their sense of a shared fate, it must signify a divergence for asymmetric partners. Ultimately all couples must embrace an essentially scientific, abstract, but highly disturbing "fact" into an everyday reality which may have been perfectly sufficient and comfortable up to that point, if they are to make the transition to safer sex. More than one individual in an ongoing asymmetric relationship mentioned that their safer sex practices were not always consistent.

Finally, a not inconsiderable issue in sexuality is the effect of illness itself. Matt stated:

> Since I have had pneumonia and my energy level dropped, I really don't have the desire for the sex. So he says it doesn't bother him, that he understands. Sometimes I think it bothers me more than it does him. (gay white male)

Gordon concurred:

> I don't think it effected us in terms of the intimacy. Frequency probably has changed because of fatigue and that has been probably the main stumbling block. (heterosexual white male)

Kaposi's sarcoma, which inflicts visible lesions, poses special problems. Tom expressed sharp disappointment at the spread of (well-camouflaged) lesions over his body:

> I have people constantly telling me: well you are still attractive, you are still fascinating, you are still personable, I could listen to you for hours, and I say, well that is all shit because when the lights go out, you are going to feel, even if you don't see them. You are going to feel bumps all over my body. (gay white man)

Bob, who was in a relationship, commented:

> There's a lot that goes along with dealing with AIDS. . . . fatigue, getting sick occasionally, having a cold and it's severe, . . . having lesions. I have a lot of them on my penis and scrotal sac, probably ten little spots and it just looks funny and I'm sure it affects a little bit how Dick feels. (gay white male)

Evan, the lover of another man with AIDS remarked:

He's lost a lot of the body and his muscle structure has deteriorated and stuff. . . . I've managed to, to kind of bring him off in a safe and gentle way a couple of times but it's hard to have sex with him in a sense that's satisfying to me. I think he knows that. I know he knows that. (gay white male)

Elsewhere in the interview, Evan reflected on the change in their relationship:

The eros was still there but it was transformed in a way to a different kind of love. I mean I would still cuddle him and hold him and all of that but it wasn't sexually charged so much as it was passionate . . . in the sense that his life was literally in immediate jeopardy and I thought he was lost and I was beginning to mourn him and have continued to mourn him. I mean I couldn't talk about this, couldn't think about this without crying. I was crying at work.

Conclusion

Perhaps some of the similarity of experiences among HIV-positive people interviewed here stems from a common lack of social and institutional support for the relationships of both homosexual men and black heterosexual women. Both groups live in social worlds which lack the community recognition, financial stability, or iconic status accorded the white middle class nuclear family, and must build relationships with few familiar guideposts to show the way. Without legal recognition, family support, or public role models, homosexual men, both black and white, accomplish long-term relationships against considerable odds. Many of the heterosexual women and men had histories of intravenous drug use and recovery, long periods of unemployment, and considerable periods of personal turmoil which also made relationship formation an uncertain venture. As Kath Weston (1991:108) remarks, gay and lesbian families show "extremely fluid boundaries, not unlike kinship organization among sectors of the African-American, American Indian, and white working class."

HIV enters into people's relationships in different ways: it poses dilemmas for single people looking for new relationships, and it forces new adjustments in ongoing relationships. Friends often also play a leading role in sorting through difficulties associated with HIV. In the early period after testing, some people with HIV infection mourn the loss of their sexuality and see that loss as part of a downward trajectory. The people we interviewed often went through a period of withdrawal from sexual activity as they sorted out issues in living with HIV infection, but, over time, took it up again.

Many people do develop new relationships. This means coming to terms with issues of disclosure of seropositivity. While in shorter-term relationships disclosure is not necessarily seen as required as long as safer sex is practiced, in ongoing relationships the issue of seropositivity arises. The most common response among these people with HIV disease is that early disclosure is generally the best policy. Potential partners often respond well to disclosure of seropositivity though HIV-positive people usually brace themselves for the worst. Indeed some respond "too well." Respondents who sought to exploit the "AIDS menace" cultural code by using their seropositivity to fend off unwanted sexual advances, sometimes found that it failed to do so.

People with HIV infection often find the responsibility for following safer sex falls on their shoulders, even when partners knew of their seropositivity. This is true, as well, in ongoing couple relationships, particularly those in which only one partner is seropositive. Couples also face the issue of changes in desire associated with states of health, raising complex issues for both ill and healthy partners.

There is sex after HIV infection and it raises a number of practical issues. These practical issues are infused with meanings that sometimes defy a "rational person" model of sexual life. Safer sex is not only a practical problem with a specific solution, but it is also a complex negotiation about love, trust, mutuality, and the erotic. Similarly, the same social codes that would demonize people with HIV infection, and cast them as the negation of desire, carry with them the obverse—the eroticization of the HIV-infected. This is not to argue that sexuality is not subject to conscious control, but rather that erotic and emotional relationships draw upon a complex interweaving of social codes, practical negotiations, and layered meanings.

Chapter Five

FAMILY AND FRIENDS

Deciding when to disclose HIV status may be a protracted issue with family and friends. Unlike lovers and spouses, who are usually told right away, less intimate relationships raise the question of appropriate timing. HIV may expose just how fragile and provisional the understandings that hold these relationships together are. Disclosure may raise previously unacknowledged aspects of one's personhood by creating a "need" to explain unknown or denied risk behaviors. HIV may act as a catalyst in exposing issues that had been suppressed or avoided, sometimes in a mutual conspiracy of silence. Still, as with domestic partners, family and friends very often rise to the occasion, and show care and resilience exceeding initial expectations.

A good deal of existing research has tried to measure these relationships in terms of the personal support available to people who are ill, and to discern the effect of support on the progress of disease—often with inconclusive results. These measures tend to hypothesize that familial relationships are, by their very nature, supportive, and that the more relationships there are, the better the patient will be, but close relationships may, of course, work either to resolve or sometimes to worsen problems associated with illness (Siegel, Raveis and Karus 1994:1555). Our

concern is to look inside existing primary relationships (as well as the
formation of new ones) to see how HIV impacts on them and how these
relationships can be part of coping with HIV. What follows are accounts
of finding one's way through relationships impacted by HIV. For both
seropositive people and caregivers, living with HIV may involve: anticipating and assessing other people's reactions, broaching the topic, and
disclosure, as well as the ways those who receive the news then sort out
issues raised by it. HIV disease, like other life-threatening diseases,
imposes a range of problems upon both ill people and their caregivers
(Wortman and Dunkel-Schetter 1979; Northouse 1984; Pearlin, Semple
and Turner 1988; Cleveland et al. 1988; Siegel and Krauss 1991; Weitz
1991; Charmaz 1991)

Care, Reliance, and "Family"

There are many scripts associated with family and intimacy which shape
expectations about giving and receiving support in times of crisis. It is
clear here that these scripts function as reference points for both people
with HIV and those in their social networks, but in practice these prescribed behaviors may be re-worked or undermined. While expectations
associated with conventional family arrangements work for some, or are
adapted to new circumstances, the people in this study display a variety
of innovative ways of creating relationships in a social field where conventional presumptions often fail to work. The family forms of lesbians
and gay men have only recently been explored in their own right apart
from traditional imputations of "deviance" and "pathology" (Levine
1991; Williams and Stafford 1991; Schneider 1992). Kath Weston
(1991:109) typifies gay and lesbian kin forms this way:

> Families we choose resembled networks in the sense that they could
> cross household lines, and both were based on ties that radiated out-
> ward from individuals like spokes on a wheel. However, gay families
> differed from networks to the extent that they quite consciously incor-
> porated symbolic demonstrations of love, shared history, material or
> emotional assistance, and other signs of enduring solidarity.

African American family forms have, as well, suffered a long tradition of
having been found wanting when measured against the nuclear family
ideals of the white middle class (Billingsley 1973). Only more recently
have they been examined to see how they do work to provide support
and survival skills for their participants. We asked people in this study to
tell us whom they cared for and relied on most, and to discuss how HIV

affected these relationships. In this way, people could identify the kinship networks that meant the most to them and talk about how their support (or its absence) mattered to them.

Sexual and affectional relationships are usually named first as the primary sources of care and support. This is clear for those in existing coupled cohabiting relationships, as well as for single people who seek them. While these stories take up most of this chapter, primary intimate relationships may also include former or nonsexual relationships.

Several gay men, both inside and outside couples, emphasize the importance of friends in their support networks. Bob said,

> But I look back at my life and all the good things that have happened and most of it is from being gay: the friendliness and the friends, the camaraderie and the family. I mean I found my outside family bigger than my inside family, my true blood family. (gay white male)

Andy concurred:

> The most important relationships in my life have been my friends and I have been very gifted in adult life 'cause I have a very, very large and close network of friends that I depend upon very heavily and they can depend on me very heavily. And no matter what crisis, I've had to come through, financial or emotional or anything, they've been there and I've been there and it'll probably continue. I have no reason to believe it would change. (gay white male)

Other gay men describe the centrality of female roommates or a heterosexual male housemate to their lives, along with siblings and parents. Tom recounted the evolution of his relationship with a friend who was to become his "buddy" appointed by an AIDS service organization:

> [At first] I did not share with him, wanting that vacation from AIDS, as it were, for a long time. . . . I hid that from him because it was nice to be with someone without having to discuss that all the time, and then when I went on the AZT, I told him, and he said he had suspected all along, and he was respecting my space. . . . [Later] he asked me if I wanted him to be my buddy, and it was absolutely perfect. We were already loving friends, and he is devoted to me, and was, he was very attracted to me. We have never been sexual, so there is still this energy . . . and I like him very much. I love him in fact. (gay white male)

The conventional division between single and coupled people, then, says little about the important relationships in these men's lives. For them, friendships carry an emotional depth which includes support, trust, and intimacy.

Telling family

Telling family members about an HIV-positive diagnosis is never easy and many agonize over the merits and timing of such a disclosure. Many people anticipate a bad family reaction. Among the participants in this study, however, a supportive response was common. Families showed a remarkable capacity to pull together and cope with the issues HIV brought home.

A number of people wanted to come to terms with testing positive before facing up to the reactions of family members. Andrea remarked:

> The only one that knows about it is my fiancé. As far as our family, we haven't told anyone. We just feel when the time is right for us to tell them we will tell them, but right now we are trying to get the best knowledge of it and get it worked out. (heterosexual black woman)

Marcia waited until after her baby was born before telling anyone of her HIV status.

> I didn't tell anyone. I was pregnant at the time. I didn't even tell my boyfriend that I had it . . . It was after I had my baby when I . . . finally told him that I had it. (heterosexual black woman)

At times, people feel they are protecting others by concealing their HIV status (Hays, Chauncey and Tobey 1990:381; Siegel and Krauss 1991). Kevin explained, "I didn't want to alarm my family, or my friend at that time." Luelle, a full-time mother living on government assistance, did not want to tell people in her family about her HIV status while her father was ill.

> I didn't tell anyone for over a year. My father had cancer real bad. He was one of the types that he was really into that sterile thing. Things had to be sterile. He had lung cancer.

She waited until after he had died to tell. Her mother already suspected that something was wrong.

> After he died, I waited for a couple of months. Then I told my mother and she took it a lot stronger than I thought she would. But like she said, she knew it was something because I guess mothers can see all. (heterosexual black woman)

For many gay men, telling family about being HIV-positive recalls an earlier process of coming out to them as gay. They often use family reactions to their coming out as a gauge of their likely response to this news they would not want to hear. Said Todd:

> I didn't really have that much fear they wouldn't accept me because they knew from a very young age that, you know, from thirteen that I was gay. . . . They were very, very supportive right from the very beginning. (gay white male)

Others who had remained closeted about their homosexuality to their families, felt that HIV would have to be treated the same way. Jason remarked:

> Since my diagnosis, though, I've kept a distance from them. I've gone to no family outings. . . . Instead of trying to justify . . . being even gay let alone HIV positive, it's better I share neither one of them with these people because it could be a hair-raising war (gay white male)

Ron anticipated this reaction from his family:

> They wouldn't look at me maliciously but they would look at me with that kind of pitying look: "Here, eat this. Make sure you gain lots of weight. Get lots of rest." . . . I am sure they would drive me crazy. (gay white male)

Sometimes delay makes disclosure increasingly difficult. Disclosure may, then, be forced by a medical crisis and happen at a time of general alarm among family members. Sheila felt she had to tell her family why she was ill.

> I was at their house because I was really sick and so like I was bullshitting to them all the whole time. I didn't want to tell them what was going on. So they were out in the waiting room when I got my results for the test, so finally after I think I was on the way home I finally had to tell my mom and dad what was going on, because they couldn't figure out why I was so sick and I was hiding stuff from them. (heterosexual white female)

In this situation, some people choose to explain their illness in terms of a different diagnosis. Fred was initially misdiagnosed as having leukemia before his HIV status became known. He continued to use this earlier diagnosis with his family.

> But I wanted to prepare them, in a way, without scaring them. So the leukemia part was the easiest part to fall back on. . . . I was not only

looking out for myself, I was looking out for them. Instead of saying, "I have got AIDS, I am not going to live," so leukemia. There was denial I think now on my part. (gay black male, previously married)

Luelle used a similar strategy for explaining the illness of her HIV infected child. The child's frequent hospital visits were explained to family members as the result of the mother's previous drug use.

But I used to use drugs and he was premature so I was always able to relate it to that, him having drugs in his system and being premature, so that worked out for a long time. But after a while that started not working too well and I still wouldn't tell. It just had to be the right time. (heterosexual black female)

Part of the reluctance to tell family members comes from the wish to avoid causing them pain, a pain incurred precisely because they care about the afflicted person. As Rick put it:

I actually feel guilt that if I die, you know, I'm thinking, oh my God, you know, how it's going to hurt my son, you know, and my girl friend and a few other people who are really close to me and that's hard—my son especially. (heterosexual white male)

Robbie had resolved to keep his HIV status to himself:

Nobody, nobody that I work with and nobody in my family knows. Nobody. All my close associates, even my gay friends, don't know. . . . I think it would hurt a lot of the family members, it would put too much pressure on them to do something or feel something, that I don't want to put them into. (gay white male)

Family members may recognize that hesitation to disclose HIV status stems from an effort to protect them from bad news. Jodi understood her brother's initial strategy of leaving town to avoid the issue of his HIV status.

His hardest time is being with the family; we've always known that. He wanted to live in Toronto so he wouldn't burden us with this . . . The guilt of this to us. (heterosexual white female)

As with other diseases, "in a troubled relationship, for example, the ill person may delay disclosing because he or she hesitates to introduce more problems into a continuing saga of conflict" (Charmaz 1991:126).

Family Responses

Though HIV-positive people frequently fear the worst, family members very often respond with sympathy and support to the disclosure. Daniel summed it up this way:

> We've had to deal with a major issue together and now we've all pulled through it, so it's brought us closer together. (gay white man)

Todd agreed:

> It has brought my sister and I closer, much closer, 'cause I've let her into my life and . . . we appreciate each other more now. (gay white man)

Rhonda found:

> A lot of people get paranoid and think that their families are going to disown them, but you would be totally surprised how much closer it brings you, because there is always that fear that they are not going to be there. (white heterosexual woman)

Daniel expressed a sentiment common among people with HIV (see Sandstrom 1990; Schwartzberg 1993:597)[1]:

> Being HIV positive, there are more benefits to me in my life from being HIV positive than if I was never diagnosed. Like I said, I'm healthier than I ever was, because I'm watching my health. I'm much more close with my family now. . . . It's strange. . . . It sounds weird but I should almost be grateful that I'm HIV positive. It's hard to say that. (gay white male)

Of course, family responses are not always so straightforward. Families may move through a series of stages in coping with HIV in one of their members (Lovejoy 1990:287; Brown and Powell-Cope 1991:339 -53). Daniel found his family was very sympathetic at first but then cooled off:

> Then . . . they just realized because I'm so healthy and everything, there's really nothing to worry about, so why do you have to be so sympathetic in the first place? They feel kind of stupid [now].

Some families have established patterns of limited or oblique styles of communication so that the disclosure of HIV status may result in only partial acknowledgement by family members (Giacquinta 1989:32). Even after Philip had told his family, he found that the subject was treated in a secretive manner:

> Nothing is mentioned in the family . . . about HIV unless my mother
> finds the miracle cure in the *Enquirer* or something. She makes sure to
> throw the article on a table where I can see it. She'll point but won't
> say anything in case someone else hears. (gay white male)

Delayed disclosure may have unanticipated costs. Frequently close family members feel betrayed at not having been told sooner about their
loved one's sero-status. In these instances, they feel upset that they had
not been trusted enough to react well to the HIV diagnosis. Not telling is
interpreted not as a concern about protecting their feelings, but as an
accusation that they would not have responded to HIV disease with care
and support. Fred worried about that problem:

> I wish they never did have to know, but I think eventually when some-
> thing does happen to me, I wouldn't want them to feel I deceived
> them by not sharing with them, because. . . . I think they will resent me
> more by not sharing it with them. . . . With Lee, my son . . . he will prob-
> ably be very angry, because I waited so long to talk to him about it. (gay
> black man)

Marcia's family found out by accident and responded this way:

> I was living with my mother at the time and I had a lot of copies [of an
> AIDS newsletter] and she went snooping in my room and found one.
> She was like, "Why didn't you tell me? You have been carrying this
> around all this time all by yourself. Girl, don't you know that we would
> have understood?" (heterosexual black woman)

Families may experience a "coming out" process once they find that one
of their members is HIV-positive. Just as the seropositive person may worry
about disclosure to family, so may family members face questions of disclosure to other relatives, neighbors, friends, and co-workers. Though a
great many gay men have been and remain involved in the daily round of
family life, their families may not have acknowledged that they are gay to
others. Indeed, apart from those who have chosen to break out of the sec-
ondary closet (and may have come to know each other through such
organizations as Parents, Friends, and Family of Lesbians and Gays,
PFLAG), many families present a conventional face to the outside world
and fail to link with other families like themselves (Frierson, Lippmann
and Johnson 1987; Cleveland et al. 1988; Stulberg and Buckingham
1988:357; Giacquinta 1989:32; Kelly and Sykes 1989:240; Bor, Miller and
Goldman 1993:191). One mother, Cindy, found that her previous
accounts of her gay son collapsed when he acquired Kaposi's sarcoma:

It makes us have to deal with it, and also, I realized I play a little game. I have three married sons. I have one single son. I play a little game and now I look like a damn fool. If you show a picture of a girl, I would say, "I have a good looking guy for her," and you play these games. So now what, now look what I have done. (heterosexual white female)

Disclosure does not always involve telling a heterosexual family. HIV-positive heterosexuals sometimes are able to turn to gay family members in the expectation that they will be more understanding. Kevin said,

My brother in Chicago, he knows I am infected. He works in a hospital so he knows different things about the disease plus he is gay so he should know a lot about it. He accepts it and asks me how I am feeling. We call each other. (heterosexual black man)

Ninia similarly counted on her gay brother-in-law:

My husband's brother is homosexual and he has been the best in the family. He comes and baby-sits for us from time to time. See, he understands it. (heterosexual white woman)

As with spouses and lovers, many found that letting family know about being HIV-positive led to a long-term deepening and strengthening of relationships. Tom reported:

If there were any gifts that came to me from all of this, it is the relationship with my father having been healed, because my father now holds me when he hugs me instead of just hugging me. (white gay man)

Jim experienced this:

It kind of opened up our relationship because for the first time—my mother raised me as a single parent—and for the first time my mother was able to speak to me as an adult on a sexual basis and for mom, that has always been hard before. (black heterosexual man)

For others, improved relationships with family members were related to having given up drug use following an HIV diagnosis. Kevin remarked:

I don't think the relationship has changed because of the disease. I think the relationship was getting more back on track because I don't use drugs. I'm sick but I don't use drugs and they like that. (heterosexual black man)

Parenting

An HIV diagnosis can pose agonizing problems for parents. Many of the seropositive parents interviewed here are African American women with histories of intravenous drug use, unemployment, and uncertain support from family or male partners. Testing HIV-positive, then, occurs in a context where the means for a basic livelihood and child care are limited or lacking altogether. Diagnosis often occurs in the context of childbearing. As Cindy Patton (1990a:102) observes,

> women almost exclusively seek testing after a male partner has been diagnosed with a symptomatic HIV syndrome, during prenatal care or after delivering a sick child, or because she has been recruited to an epidemiologic study. . . . Thus, women's knowledge of serostatus precedes their realization that they might be at risk. . . . For the most part, women have difficulty perceiving themselves as "at risk" because they view themselves as engaging in "ordinary" or "normal" and therefore "safe" heterosexual intercourse.

Coping with the news of one's own diagnosis may soon be followed by many anxious months of waiting for a diagnosis of a newborn child whose sero-status may not become clear until the child's immune system begins to form antibodies of its own. Many women then enter into a troubled relationship with social service agencies in their search for the resources to provide for themselves and for their children. While child care is often difficult to secure in the best of times, some women reported that child care agencies exclude their children on the grounds that they would not take legal responsibility for administering medication to them. Their children's need for frequent and regular doses of AZT made them impossible to place. Crystal found that child care workers refused to change her child's diaper and wanted to remove him from the other children:

> They had him in a little jail, a play pen, where he had to stay. . . . This one little girl wanted to get in the play pen with him to play with Michael but they wouldn't allow it. They wouldn't let Michael out. They wouldn't let Jessica in. (heterosexual black woman)

While the women's needs became more acute in the context of HIV disease, they also became more fearful of dealing with social service agencies who tended to view their personal histories, in combination with their sero-status, as reason to label them unfit mothers. At the moment when their need for basic services was greatest, they felt at greatest risk of losing their children and so tended to avoid social service offices.[2] In Crystal's words:

A lot of women don't want help because they are scared that the city or whoever takes the baby from people. . . . They feel as though once those child protective workers get on your case, if you use [drugs] and you are HIV [positive], that they will snatch up your child.

For women who have been through this process and have older children, the problems may not get any easier. Ninia said,

I got pregnant with him when I was 16. I was very irresponsible; I tried keeping him but I couldn't. He has been through foster homes, and social services, and children's homes because I couldn't get myself together. I was running the streets. I certainly couldn't look after a child and he has been with me on and off. They would let him come home, and then I would screw up and they would take him away. . . . When I started to get my life together, I started getting in touch with . . . my son. My son and I are building a relationship. He has told me he has a lot of anger towards me. . . . and we have been to therapy with him. (heterosexual white woman)

Noncustodial parents may face the problem of explaining HIV to their children amidst an already troubled family dynamic. Noncustodial parents may fear that their HIV status could become a weapon used by their ex-spouses to malign them to their children, or to curtail or prevent access to them. As well, being the absent parent increases the difficulty of expressing painful news to children. Elizabeth, the fiancée of a seropositive man remarked that his son is:

still really uncomfortable about acknowledging that his dad has AIDS and that is partly because he doesn't really understand it. . . . partially because of his mother because his mother won't, and partially because of his age [13]. (heterosexual white woman)

Telling children may also raise a problem of explaining one's risk status, as it does with other audiences. Robbie explains,

I have two children, and one is in high school and they certainly are not stupid about being gay and that sort of thing, but they do not know my lifestyle. And, uh, if I told them that I was positive then their mother, my ex-wife, would make sure I would not see them. She has this built up fear that you can gain it by, you know, osmosis I guess. . . . That's my biggest problem right now, is what to do about them. . . . The worst thing is being separated from my children. (gay white man)

Nick struggled over similar issues:

There are many people out there who are HIV positive who are married with children. I am one of them. And it is a very difficult issue to deal with. I don't know how to handle it, so I don't handle it. . . . I want them to know who I am and this is part of who I am. But I can't do it. . . . They know I am gay. They know I am a homosexual. My ex-wife knows I am a homosexual, but that is not an issue, but this [seropositivity] is for me. And I know there are other people out there who have children of all ages, and it is a problem for them too, but none of us have had an answer. (gay white male)

Finding one's parents to be HIV-positive may be an overwhelming experience for young children, especially when both parents are affected. Gordon comments on his daughter of primary school age:

She was terrified on a couple of occasions when I wasn't feeling well and [wife] wasn't feeling well with other things, that this was AIDS and you were going to die. And it took a lot of time to explain. . . . because I think initially . . . she understood but she didn't believe it. . . . There was a long period where she was very concerned since both of us had it, the both of us could be dying and she could be sort of on her own. . . . It was hard for her, because on one hand she nodded her head and said, "I believe what you are telling me," and then on the other hand I don't think she believed a word. She just knew that she could be left without anybody. (heterosexual white male)

For older children, disclosure may be similar to telling other adults. Kevin found:

My son has known . . . since the time that I was in the prison hospital. At the time he was a senior in high school; he had just finished high school. He was like 17 but, I always raised him to be open minded. He is intelligent, he understands the disease, not the plague. He doesn't have any problems dealing with it. He hates to see me sick, but he understands. (black heterosexual man)

The Unsupportive Family

People in this study commonly received a supportive response from their family members when they disclosed their HIV-positivity. There are some families, however, who react badly, especially those who found out in the period of 1985 to 1987 at the height of the AIDS hysteria in North America. In these instances, family members asked their HIV-positive kin to eat from separate plates or to keep away from their nieces and nephews. Wally lived with his father for a month:

I spent my nights on the couch. . . . He took away the remote control because . . . I was touching it with my dirty hands and he would put the cover over the couch. When I moved out, he gave me the sheets. . . . He was just damned scared. (white heterosexual man)

Sheila experienced similar treatment:

So they are OK about it, but first my mom was like, I know one night I freaked out on her because, I felt like she was treating me like I had the plague—make sure I put my glass in the dishwasher when I am done. Do this and do that. She wouldn't even let me eat out of the same bag of chips as my brother. Like I was freaked on her, I said, "You can't get it from eating out of the same bag of frickin chips you know." So she sent away in *Woman's Day* some literature and started reading on it, so she is OK about it now. (white heterosexual woman)

The negative message of family "quarantine" counteracts positive words. Bill found that his mother implemented a quarantine that implied she held him responsible for his condition.

The first night when I told them, they were very parenting, sympathetic, "Just go on with your daily life and live and take care of business" like. But it was my mother, "Go about your business like you normally do"—this is what her lips said, but the next day her actions and everything else said something totally different. Paper plates came out of the cabinets and the plastic forks and here is your paper cup and here is your special cup to drink out of, and she was so nervous she would walk around the house, and if I would go into the kitchen, she would come to see what I was touching. She would come in there to make inspections. Then she told me a week later, "I don't want any of my children to catch what you have got. You had a choice in the matter and they don't have a choice." (gay black man)

Six people we talked to complained of some sort of quarantine in the homes of others, particularly family members. This kind of experience was common to all kinds of HIV-positive people regardless of whether they are women or men; gay, straight, or bisexual; drug users or non-users; or black or white. Quarantine sends a strong negative message; on the other hand, such actions as sharing food and dishes can be read as a true sign of loyalty and support. Rhonda said, "but they still love me, they will take a bite of my sandwich after I have and things" (heterosexual white female).

As in the instance of Bill's mother, an HIV diagnosis may be the occasion for the reassertion of homophobia that may have been previously assuaged among family members (Rowe, Plum and Crossman 1988:77;

Weitz 1989:105; Cates et al. 1990:198). Devon found that his family condemned him while he was lying in bed in hospital, saying they always believed that his homosexuality was wrong.

> They came in and they marched in in a single file waiting to condemn me, and they condemned me. . . . I was very frustrated with that and I called the nurse and I had every last one of them put out. There were six or seven of them, my family members. (gay black male)

Marcia avoided telling her family of her HIV-status because of their earlier rejection of her drug use, like the gay men who anticipated their family's reaction based on (lack of) acceptance of their risk status.

> I wasn't going to tell them. I was already the black sheep of the family because I use drugs. I wasn't going to tell them, because I know it would have been a lot of rejection, but I just deal with it. I just kept it to myself. It was like a heavy burden for me. I was carrying around a heavy burden. (heterosexual black woman)

Even among supportive families, there may be one family member who holds out against the others (Weitz 1991:105). The sister of Peter's sister-in-law disputed how to respond to his diagnosis:

> One sister said, "Well I don't want her coming to my house any more because she might have germs on her that my little girl could catch from, you know, living with that guy with AIDS." And so she has not spoke to her one sister. . . . so they're real paranoid. (white gay man)

Double Disclosure

For some, disclosure of HIV status also raises the problem of discussing previously undisclosed behaviors. Sometimes this means bringing up homosexuality to a wife or drug use to parents. This dilemma convinces some people to avoid situations where the double disclosure might come up (Wolcott et al. 1986:399). Managing information about HIV, however, cannot always be pulled off. Tony's parents found out only when he was hospitalized with PCP. He says,

> I don't know exactly how they found out. . . . I remember they came in and once I was conscious they . . . talked to me, "So we know what you have and it is OK and we still love you. We will be here for you." And they always have been quite wonderful. I didn't want it to get to that point. I always wanted to tell them before then because of the double whammy. (gay white man)

Jim remarked:

> At the time I told my wife, my fiancée, I told her about me having experienced being with a man before and so this was the first time this subject had even come into the light. She didn't have any suspicion or inclination so it was kind of hard to deal with. (heterosexual black male)

His fiancée responded by confessing to another relationship she had had while he had been incarcerated. He concluded:

> I don't really regret it too much because it has helped me find who I am and it has helped me and her have a better understanding of her sexuality, her practices, and mine. I think we love each other a little bit more because of it.

Tony also experienced the relief of having "come out of the closet" after giving his family the "double whammy":

> I feel closer to my parents than I did before. It has taken a lot of burden off me too. Finally they know. There is no big secret we have to talk around all the time. . . . I can actually say what I am doing instead of pretending that I am going to a movie with a friend. (gay white man)

Carl was pleasantly surprised when his disclosure worked out well.

> My family dealt with it real well, which I was real surprised. My parents had just got divorced. I didn't know what to do. My father and I were really not that close and he was very macho and first he has got to learn that he has a gay son. He didn't know that. He didn't know for sure— this definitely put a damper on things. He was there everyday, supportive, still is supportive and he really helps. Even when you think your family and people are not going to react in a good way, you just don't know them good enough sometimes. (gay white male)

Of course the double revelation can have unpredictable results. Said Matt:

> I always thought he [brother] would be a real red neck and when I told him I was gay, he says, "That's OK. I tried it but it wasn't for me." He shocked me more than I shocked him! (gay white male)

People who were not gay or drug users did not have to go through the same double disclosure. They did, however, have to deal with the fact that the people they told identified HIV infection with gay people or drug users. Paula found that her family strongly associated HIV infection with certain groups.

They took it as a shock. People expect gay people to have it, not people like me that don't use drugs, or was a prostitute, or anything like that. (heterosexual black woman)

In-Law Relations

Relationships with in-laws have a legendary reputation of requiring diplomatic skills and special care, as they lack the easy familiarity common among blood ties. Almost nothing has been written of the relationships between same-sex partners and their in-law equivalents (but see Denneny 1979). Yet despite a widespread public discourse that opposes homosexual men to "the family," most are actively engaged in family relationships which include affines along with biological kin. As with so many other social relationships, HIV may act as a catalyst in exposing underlying questions and tensions. A not uncommon "arrangement" among families with gay members is a fragile unspoken agreement that the same-sex relationship will remain formally unacknowledged and unspoken, though "everybody knows." HIV may also be enclosed by this closet strategy where illness is denied and the denial is, in turn, denied as well (see Sedgwick 1990). Alexander remarked of his lover of two years:

His family doesn't know about his disease. They don't really know officially about him being gay, except that they know me. So they don't know—they are very intelligent people—they don't know about his disease. (gay white male)

Some families may resist ever acknowledging a gay relationship (Land and Harangody 1990:477), but over time, the keeping up of pretenses may break down. Leo described it this way:

I know that he talks about me when he goes over. When his parents call him, they ask about me, what I am doing. They are coming around. It took a while though. They knew he was gay and had to have a relationship with a man, but I think they didn't want to hear about it. (gay white male)

Doug found that over time the illness of his partner brought him closer to his partner's mother:

We had to because she was giving me calls, you know. I'm working nights at work and I'm getting calls, "I don't know what to do with Bruce. He's threatening to kill himself. He's going to pop all these pills," and everything else like that. I'd get her to calm down. . . . So, after dealing with all these incidents, . . . we got closer. (gay white male)

Evan, a white professional man, describes a lengthy process of rapprochement with the family of his black lover of five years:

I think his mother thought it was very high-handed of me to get his power of attorney and go around, you know, in my suit, acting on his behalf, threatening people and basically making a general nuisance of myself because I think she thought, you know, doctors are going [to] take care of him and I think that was a bad assumption. . . . I'd come in the house and stuff but they kind of kept me in the outer parlor. . . . Here, I'm showing up there as the lover of their son, right? So there was a little bit of distance certainly. . . . When he's been hospitalized which is now four times for lengthy periods, we share, without even saying anything, we share the time we spend with him. It's like, I say, "Are you going down at lunch?" "Yeah, I'll be there at lunch." "Will you be there at supper?" "Right." "What are you bringing?" "I'll bring this," and it's like I'm a member of their family as far as that's concerned. (gay white male)

Anne, the lesbian caregiver to Sheila, a heterosexual woman, did not expect a favorable response from the latter's family. Indeed, the anticipated response became a joke among them. She now assumes that the parents have figured out the relationship and accept it on the basis that they are helpful to Sheila.

We joked to Sheila, "Oh well, wait till you tell her that I am gay," and we would laugh about it. But I think actually her parents know that Deborah and I are lovers, but we are such a positive atmosphere and influence around her that that is what is important to them.

Same-sex partners and other-sex spouses may both receive flak from their own families for staying with their HIV-positive partner. Linda encountered these reactions from her family:

My sister said, "What are you nuts?" and the only nonjudging person is my mother. I'm sure she is, but she doesn't show it, and my one sister— I have three—won't let us in her house. Her husband says we can't come over. (heterosexual white female)

Evan also had to deal with his sister's advice:

I'm close to my sister and I told her and she was horrified for me and . . . I said, "I don't think you're listening. What I'm suffering now is a

threat to my friend. I'm not that worried about me." And she tried to
hector me and lecture me about, "Oh Evan, you don't know how to
choose partners anyway. I never did like him anyway." (gay white male)

These kinds of troubled relationships may explain the findings of
Robert Hays, Sarah Chauncey, and Linda Tobey (1990:381) that "networks composed predominantly of peers were associated with greater
psychological well-being than networks containing high percentages of
relatives" for people living with HIV disease, a finding confirmed by
other researchers (McCann and Wadsworth 1992; Britton, Zarski and
Hobfoll 1993).

Telling friends

Initial disclosures may be made to other people who are HIV-positive
themselves. Gay men may tell gay friends first on the presumption that
they will be well acquainted with and sympathetic to having HIV. Robbie
told his lover and a few other people.

> I told my neighbor downstairs who is also gay, who had a friend, a very
> close friend, that died last year, so he was very sensitive to the whole
> thing. I felt safe to talk to him. And one of the fellows involved with the
> PWA support group . . . is a personal friend of mine, so I talked to him.
> That was it. (gay white male)

Gregory explained that the shared experience of HIV could be an important source of support.

> We both cried together. He helped me out. He explained as much as
> he could, but maybe because he also had a friend who had AIDS or actu-
> ally a relative. That made me feel a lot better inside. (gay white male)

Todd found it very important to have HIV positive friends with him to
share the experience.

> I started meeting a lot of other people [with AIDS] from here and
> Toronto that are now five, six, seven, eight years and with that, you
> know, it really helped to turn it over . . . It's not automatically a death
> sentence; something I've learned to live with. (gay white male)

Friends may have their own anxieties to deal with after being told.
Finding out about HIV in a friend may lead people to confront more
directly their own vulnerability to AIDS. Ron described the way his
friends responded:

The first reaction was shock, through my gay male friends, a lot of them it really rocked because I was never much of a slut, so to speak, and . . . some of them were a lot more guilty than I am, yet afraid to take the test. None of them had been tested. A lot of their reaction was, "Why did you get tested? What did you bother for?"—strict denial. But they have all been very supportive. I haven't had one friend skip out on me from knowing and after a little adjustment period we are right back to normal. (gay white male)

Sometimes talking with friends may happen with an ease that escapes sexual or familial relationships. Anne, the friend of a seropositive woman, remarks,

It opened up our communication door even wider, and it just sort of advanced it quicker. We got close faster because of it, but I think we would have ended up going in that path anyway. (white lesbian)

People who had been through recovery programs often disclosed to counselors or support groups connected to recovery. Sheila found some support within her recovery support groups:

Like a few people know, like people that I am in the program with, NA and AA. And like I trust them, so there are maybe six people that know. Just talking to them, I guess after a while I wasn't dying and I am getting better, so I figured maybe that is not the way it is. (heterosexual white female)

There are certain situations in which people do not want to take a chance with the reaction of others. In prison, for example, letting others know your HIV status can be dangerous. Kevin, who found out he was HIV positive in prison did not talk about it with others.

And by being in prison is not something that you want to discuss with people, because you don't really get that close to anyone, at least I didn't. And if I did discuss it with anyone they would spread it over the population and I would have problems. So the only person I ever spoke to about it was the psychiatric nurse and she didn't have too much information. (black heterosexual man)

Jim, who also found out in prison, carefully selected a fellow inmate to confide in and found it very helpful.

He was telling me about polio when he was a kid, used to kill a lot of people. He told me just to keep my head up, not to be down, so he kind of cheered me up while I was in there. (black heterosexual man)

Indeed, having someone to talk to could be a major reason for joining an HIV support group. As Marcia said,

> I didn't want to be bothered because I don't want to go around and sit with a bunch of people who got AIDS. I was already in a state of denial myself. . . . So the lady just kept bugging me and bugging me, so I just told her "Yeah, I'm a coming" and that Wednesday I came. So I went that one time and I just loved that support group. There was so much love there and a lot of support. Everybody care for each other. And it helps me to deal with life from day to day and it just gives me a lot of strength. It's my strength. (black heterosexual woman)

Conclusion

HIV can disrupt understandings built up over many years among friends and family members. While most families and friends are able to deepen mutual ties in the face of HIV, some relationships unravel to reveal underlying homophobia or distrust. Telling dependent children is especially difficult. Custodial parents worry about assuaging children's fears of abandonment at the same time as they are dealing with their own sense of mortality. Even as seropositive mothers are attempting to provide for their children against tremendous odds even at the best of times, HIV imposes yet another overwhelming demand in trying to secure their futures. Noncustodial parents, whether black or white, male or female, gay or heterosexual, feel troubled by the prospect that HIV can be used against them by their spouses to block access to their children, at a time when they feel most emotionally vulnerable and want the time they have to be spent with those they most care about.

These interviews also offer a glimpse into the relationships which gay men have with their lovers' families, a topic almost entirely ignored in the research literature and denied by popular ideologies which conceive of lesbians and gay men as a species opposed to "the family" and everyday life. An unacknowledged yet pervasive secret in our society is the ways in which gay people are, in fact, integrated into the daily rounds of family life, a denial institutionalized in law and official discourse.

Among the many effects of chronic disease on caregivers in general, Juliet Corbin and Anselm Strauss (1988:293; see also Charmaz 1991) list the following salient issues:

> (1) conflict over control of illness management, (2) constancy of the work and the resource drain it brings about, (3) feeling the burden of three lines of work, (4) spouse overload . . . , (5) juggling of the needs

of the ill person with the spouse's biographical needs, (6) sexual frustration, (7) anxiety over dwindling financial resources, (8) fear of dying, (9) feelings of isolation and loneliness, (10) biographical disruption and biographical limbo, and (11) change in the nature of the marital relationships (including a spouse's resentment) and lack of a mutually sustaining relationship.

When one member of a gay couple becomes ill with HIV disease, a range of responsibilities falls to the well partner:

> running the household, providing nursing care to the person with AIDS, managing finances and legal matters, participating in medical decisions and serving as a liaison between the person with AIDS and his or her social network (Maj 1991:162; see also Brown and Powell-Cope 1991:339).

The ways in which caregivers live with HIV in their own ways tend to go unrecognized. Doug noted:

> I never really, uh, went to anyone for support. I was more or less going around looking for someone for support for him. . . . One of the things that really bothers me, . . . [is] it's never very much for, okay, "Let's figure out how we can help the caregiver." You don't have that happen. People who have gone through it will come up to me and say, "How are you doing?" They'll know what it's like and everything. (gay white male)

Other caregivers caution against neglecting one's own well-being while taking care of the needs of the person with HIV. Evan recommends to other caregivers:

> Think of your own resources, your own emotional resources, even physical resources. Don't push yourself past the limit because you'll overreact. Try to keep a level head and try to keep your own work in perspective and don't try to be Florence Nightingale. (gay white male)

Or in Dino's words:

> Confront it as honestly and openly as you would anything else. Be a friend; don't be a doormat. Get support in support groups. I think that's important. And finally, just take it one day at a time. (gay white male)

Chapter Six

WORKING

HIV infection creates a number of dilemmas around employment. As with friends and family, HIV status may need to be revealed to managers and co-workers, especially when symptoms interfere with the ability to perform one's job. Despite legislation in both the United States and Canada which protects people with HIV from discrimination due to disability, HIV infection may be used by employers to deprive people of their livelihood, even when they are fully capable of continuing on the job. Of course, loss of a job almost always results in financial insecurity and for many people, the erosion of their independence and sense of self-worth. Though the issues around AIDS and work are commonly conceptualized in terms of withdrawal from the labor market, many HIV-positive people are just starting careers or are looking for employment, as they are able and willing to work. Some hope that seropositivity may provide them with new opportunities in the AIDS "industry" as safe-sex educators or agency staff.

The participants in this study range from a senior administrator with a large corporation to people who have spent years on the margins of paid employment in domestic labor and in welfare systems. At the time of the interview, most participants had low incomes, with 35 living on less than $10,000 per year, 22 on more.[1] This low income figure reflects the fact that 37 of the 60 participants were not employed. At least 23 of the 37 had stopped working, whether voluntarily or involuntarily, since testing HIV positive. The low income figures also reflect the class and occupational status of these respondents. Twenty work in white collar jobs such as social service work, teaching, computer programming, or design. Fifteen work in service jobs such as waiting tables or retail sales, of whom four are in part-time or casual positions. Eight work in clerical jobs. Four are in factory or transportation work. One respondent is a corporate executive. Twelve did not describe an occupation, seven because of long-term absence from the labor market, while three were full-time parents, and two were students.

The existing research literature on AIDS and the workplace has generally avoided the *experiences* of people with HIV disease. Rather, it begins with an organizational point of view, casting seropositive people as a problem for the smooth functioning of corporations.[2] In the words of Alan Emery and Sam Puckett (1988:3), books on AIDS and work typically address "managers who are concerned about managing the consequences of this epidemic in the workplace." An assumption of the organizational literature is that people with HIV should be hired and kept employed provided that they *can do the job*, either their own or an alternative within the organization (see Patterson 1989:40). When a person ceases to be able to meet production norms, it is taken for granted by organizational theory that their employment will cease, hopefully in the way that is least disruptive for all concerned. What is missing from this approach is a concern for the overall well-being of workers as viewed from the workers' perspective. Work may be expected to fulfill a range of needs, including economic survival with a decent standard of living, job satisfaction, and finding a place in the world (Lebowitz 1992:56). The focus here is to understand the challenges that work or joblessness pose from the viewpoint of people with HIV infection.

The workplace, then, presents a number of challenges to be negotiated by people living with HIV. The ability and the right to work may come into dispute. Employers will often not tolerate or compensate for the intrusion of such "private" issues as sickness, sexuality, drug use, or grieving into the workplace. Job loss can lead to a precipitous decline in standard of living and quality of life, particularly in the United States where workplace benefit plans are crucial for access to medical services. The economic decline associated with job loss is compounded by a popular tendency to measure people in terms of their place in the labor market (see Fox 1980). Thus, joblessness can often be equated with lack of worth, whether by self or others. Given the dominant sexual division of labor, this is bound to be particularly true for men, though it is increasingly true for women as well. Some people with HIV solve work-related problems by withdrawing from paid employment, while others continue in their jobs and develop strategies for handling them. This chapter examines the problems of the workplace and the creative measures developed to deal with them.

Looking for Work

HIV is not a one-way street out of the job market. Some of the people we interviewed were actively looking for work or engaged in education toward a future career. Their job searches were particularly difficult due to the recession of the early 1990s. Wayne described these difficult circumstances.

> I was going on interviews. I still am, but I don't know why. I'm not getting—oh, Michigan has slacked off quite a bit. (gay white male)

Some participants say that getting a job, or education toward a career, is part of a process of changing their lives for the better in response to HIV. This is particularly true of people who had been outside of the conventional job market for extended periods of time, often because of the absence of employment opportunities or of drug use and related issues. Jim is a former drug user who had been in prison and had plans to go to school.

> I plan to be in school for a while. I want to get a paralegal certification, so before I go to law school, because of my prison record, I think that would be a plus. So I want to kind of turn things around, just make that little extra effort, to show the particular law school anyway that I have tried to, to do the best that I can. (bisexual black male).

Securing a job can be complicated by the difficulty in finding child care, drug-related gaps in employment history, and a limited job market. Marcia also raised the issue of disclosing her HIV status to potential employers.

> The papers that you have to fill out for a job, they ask you about your medical history and stuff, so I am dealing with: I have to lie or what? (heterosexual black female)

Andrea expressed concern about workplace drug testing and the possibility of HIV testing. She had resolved not to disclose her HIV-status in a potential employment situation.

The only thing that I could say is a lot of times, they is doing these blood, they doing urine tests for drugs. They do the drug testing 'fore you come on duty, and if they tested me for HIV, I could see a problem there. When I fill out the form it is going to be, "No, No, No." . . . I am not going to stop myself from getting anything before I can get it. (heterosexual black female)

Two respondents expressed concern about working in particular occupations given their HIV status. Marcia was unsure if she should work in the field for which she was trained as it involves direct contact with blood.

I am a certified phlebotomist, and I am not employed right now because I am still trying to deal with if it is right for me, going through with this work, and I am HIV infected. A phlebotomist is where you draw blood. (heterosexual black female)

Jordan expressed concern about working in a restaurant, despite the absence of any actual public health threat.

I don't know, sometimes I don't think it has any impact. Sometime if you are working in a place like a restaurant, you have a tendency to worry about whether or not you are going to cut yourself and splatter blood all over the food or plates. That might make you a little self-conscious about it. I used to work in a restaurant before HIV. (bisexual black male).

Others, who disliked their current jobs or had not found a career path, hoped to turn HIV into an asset in seeking employment in AIDS service organizations.

Staying at Work

While the advice literature on AIDS and the workplace recommends cooperative problem solving, it is an ideal that is seldom realized. James Nichols writes, "Like work, AIDS takes place in the context of personal relationships. It needs to be co-managed not managed" (Tedlow and Marram 1991:15). Although there are some examples of successful co-management among the participants in this study, the nature of workplace control in capitalist societies constrains the development of trust in management, or confidence in equitable treatment, that would be required for genuine co-management. If a few cautious generalizations can be offered based on the experiences of HIV-positive workers in this study, it is that workers fare better when they have gay supervisors, in small organizations characterized by personal, face-to-face relations with managers, and conversely, in large organizations with formal policies mandating the treatment of AIDS issues. Workers without the protection of law or union regulation are otherwise left to the preconceptions and arbitrary actions of individual employers. Duane described his workplace as "a nightmare."

> I'm a fighter. I fought five landlords, God knows how many employers. I'm a fighter. I fight this virus, but I've had, for me the closest thing to a nightmare, in terms of the workplace. It is very difficult. (gay white male)

The relative powerlessness of workers leads many to conclude that disclosure of their HIV status is simply too risky. Nick reasoned this way.

> I don't want to do anything to jeopardize that, because I really enjoy it. And I don't know what might happen, so rather then create a situation that I have no idea what the outcome will be, I would rather deal with it and keep my work as long as possible without causing controversy, without exposing myself to a whole host of things. . . . So I keep myself quiet about my personal life and my personal status. (gay white male)

Not all employers and supervisors react badly; indeed, many respond with decency and compassion well beyond the call of duty. Nonetheless, many people with HIV infection envision their workplace responses as a worst-case scenario to avoid risking everything and hoping for the best. A number of participants told us about supportive employers. Some were quite pleasantly surprised by their supervisors. Peter first spoke to his supervisor when he thought he had leukemia and then spoke to him again when he found out it was HIV infection. Not only had his supervisor anticipated the news, but he was also quite knowledgeable about HIV.

> He [supervisor] said, "Because after I found out it wasn't leukemia, this was probably the next ultimate choice it could be so I did some research on that" and he was really more informed at that point than I was. (gay white male)

This supervisor was so committed to keeping this employee on that he was willing to overlook problems in work performance:

> My boss was very understanding, thank God. He was really wonderful [concerning dementia]. Even after my diagnosis, when I told him, he didn't want me to quit. He didn't want me to leave and I was making some real serious mistakes. I made one mistake which cost us $2300 in one day.

Carl expected his employer to respond well, as he worked in hairdressing, an occupation with a lot of gay workers affected by the AIDS epidemic.

> Everybody that I can think of knows about me. . . . They've been totally supportive and there you go, they'll eat off your plate, things that you would be just totally amazed. They were prepared, but we had someone already die of AIDS, that worked there at the salon. They were not unaware, hairdressers. You're labeling yourself. Look at where AIDS has hit most is in the fashion industry, hairdressing. Where are gays most effective? So of course they're going to hear about it. (gay white male)

When Barb re-entered the workforce, she chose to work for a particular employer because of her previous good experience in disclosing her seropositivity to him.

> Part of it was because my daughter was still not school age and I needed to have the flexibility. The other part could very well have been that he was a safe person and he already knew. He wasn't going to ask me any questions. (heterosexual white/aboriginal female)

While some individuals met with generous and creative responses to their seropositivity, Chad did not.

> And I thought I had cancer and I was running around work telling people I was dying of cancer. I don't know why I was doing that. So my boss, the owner of the restaurant grabbed me . . . by the shirt collar and said, "If you have fucking AIDS I don't want you in my fucking restaurant. If you have fucking AIDS I can't afford to lose my business. You get the hell out of here" and stuff. It just threw me for a big one. I went, "No, there is nothing wrong with me. I am just being neurotic" and that was that, and I denied everything, and got myself out of it. I am a very good actor when I have to be. (gay white male)

Duane was told to stop his habit of bringing in special treats for other workers to share:

> I was told, don't bring any foodstuffs in. I was told that specifically. I was brought aside by the owner of the business. He said, "I don't know why you bring these in. We don't want them." I said, "Fine, I'm not going to spend the money." (gay white male)

People with HIV have to weigh many factors in developing a strategy for handling their HIV-status at work. Co-management works at times but only a few have the luxury of being able to anticipate an understanding response from their employers. There is no guarantee of compassion. Fundamental power inequalities structure the workplace, laying the grounds for generosity and creativity, or for harassment, humiliation, or dismissal.

Telling People at Work

A central issue that people with HIV face in the workplace is disclosure. People must decide whether or not to inform others of their HIV status. Nondisclosure reduces the risk of discriminatory action, but disclosure may provide an acceptable explanation for changes in work practices or performance. Not telling may be relatively easy for someone who is completely healthy, but people who face HIV-related health problems are obliged to give some account of themselves. People living with other chronic illnesses often face similar dilemmas. Scambler (1984:216) reports that most people with epilepsy adopt a strategy of concealment at work, disclosing only when it cannot be avoided. Robbie adopted a blanket policy of nondisclosure.

> Nobody, nobody that I work with and nobody in my family knows. Nobody. All my close associates, even my gay friends, don't know. It's like business as usual. (gay white male)

Not telling can reduce risks, though it may be difficult to negotiate. Joe weighed some of the potential advantages of disclosure against the risks, and decided he would rather leave his teaching job than disclose his HIV-status.

> Sometimes I would like to tell somebody in administration, just in case I was having a problem, a health problem, because we need to keep in mind that I have been off work for a whole year. . . . There are some guidelines, but I don't know to what extent they have been exercised. I would rather just not chance it. (bisexual black male).

Other people choose to discuss their HIV status with carefully selected people at work. Gordon remarked,

> For me it was easier after a year or so of trying to keep them at bay, saying, "Look, I am HIV positive. You have always known I was a hemophiliac. Here is the situation." (heterosexual white male).

Tony chose to tell a close friend and gay people at work, trusting that they could deal with AIDS issues. He told,

A real close female friend that I work pretty closely with. She knows and then there are a couple other gay people. Yeah the one gay guy who is in management, I guess, a boss—he is not my boss, he is a friend too—so I told him, and I told everybody that knows. I am sure if it was general knowledge that I would have a lot more problems. (gay white male)

Matt worked for a district manager who knew his HIV-status through connections in the gay community:

My district manager knows, but then he is gay, so it's not a problem there. . . . He knew I was positive when they hired me. I was up for a promotion at work and he turned me down for it because it would have put me out of his jurisdiction. That way he wanted me in his jurisdiction. That way if there was a problem, like needing off work, he could deal with it, where if he let me go out of his area, he would have no control over it. (gay white male)

The issue of disclosure is often closely linked to coming out as gay. A network of gay or gay-positive individuals in the workplace can provide support for handling issues of sexuality and seropositivity. Disclosing seropositivity at work may be safer for people who do not have to announce their membership in a stigmatized minority at the same time.

Even so, some people took the risk because they felt there were specific work-related reasons to disclose. Jeff is a nurse who wanted the right to refuse certain patients who posed a potential health risk to him.

I informed my superior, my charge nurse. She didn't have to know . . . but I told her anyway so she would understand why I would refuse to take certain patients, for example, whooping cough. . . . [The reaction at work] was very good. I was an openly gay individual but I didn't push it on anybody. (gay white/aboriginal male)

In contrast to this deliberate strategy of disclosure for work-related reasons, Tom told his supervisor out of exasperation. He was in senior management of a large corporation and therefore able to act with more confidence than many other respondents.

So my supervisor reported to the vice president. It was like telling the world and being a huge risk and she was a woman with whom I did not feel great trust . . . and I simply went in one day and said, "I am unwilling to continue being here under these circumstances any longer, that is, that I drag my butt in here and I don't get acknowledgement for what has been going on and one of the things that happened is that

> when I had shingles, I came in here and you, instead of asking me in
> a delicate, gentle, inquiring way, 'What is wrong with your hand?' even
> though you had seen me around the office, and might have heard
> other people talking that there was something wrong with me, you
> said, 'Oh! What's that?' " and I said, "That reaction is not acceptable
> to me, completely unacceptable. What that is is shingles and it may or
> may not be related to the fact that I have been tested and I am a posi-
> tive to the virus and it is impacting on my job and I feel that you as my
> supervisor have a right to know that this is one of the things that I am
> dealing with in my life and that is the communication." She said, "Well
> thank you for telling me" and that was that issue. (gay white male)

The supervisor took the disclosure well, but others are not so fortunate. Daniel said disclosure to his supervisor harmed their working
relationship.

> I did tell my manager, which was kind of a mistake, I think. I didn't
> know any better at the time. That's when I was calling in sick and stuff
> so finally I said I've got to tell her. We sat down together and I said,
> "You know, there's something I've got to tell you. I just tested positive
> for the AIDS virus" and she was kind of shocked. I got her a whole
> bunch of pamphlets from the AIDS Committee and stuff . . . but I think
> that she, it scared her a lot, and I think her attitude about me com-
> pletely changed. . . . She lost some respect for me and, you know, the
> typical straight person who blames gays for a lot of things and she was
> doing that a little with me. (gay white male)

Perhaps the most worrisome situation is a leak which exposes HIV-status
to an employer. Though ruptures in medical confidentiality may be
unethical and even illegal, procedures for redress may be too cumbersome or taxing to follow. A doctor exposed Devon when he needed a
note to cover a failure to respond to his beeper.

> I wasn't able to answer my beeper so I was out for a few days afterwards
> although we had made contact, but in order for me to come back to
> work they needed some type of documentation stating where I was
> when I was beeped. So my doctor, not thinking, sent my entire med-
> ical record to my director, who was a [nurse], and it had HIV written all
> over it. (gay black male)

When health insurance is employment-related, it may be difficult to
ensure that information about medical treatment will not spill over into
the workplace. Evan expressed concern that medical bills going to his
employer might reveal his history of testing for HIV-related conditions.

So the people in the accounting department and whoever handle benefits in that building know that I've been interested in my HIV status for a long time. . . . I was thinking to myself, well, somehow that was going to be part of my employment record. (gay white male)

Working vs Illness

HIV infection may impair physical or mental abilities to do certain kinds of work. It may then become necessary to refuse certain kinds of work, to require more sick days, or to cope with fatigue. Any of these may be defined by employers as a failure to do the job. Fred left a job that he defined as too physically demanding.

> Then I started having trouble with my leg. It is still swollen. They are in the process of working on that and it got so that I really couldn't work, because I encountered a lot of walking, a lot of standing. I just couldn't do it. (gay black male)

Gregory tried to avoid work that demanded physical exertion.

> Sometimes, particularly jobs I feel I can't do, like heavy lifting, I just seem to disintegrate when I am doing really hard work. So I try to find something that is not too hard on myself, or whatever. (gay white male)

Edward Yelin, et al. (1991:83) argue that people with HIV whose work requires high physical exertion, and who have less control over the pace of work, are more likely to have to withdraw from employment. Joe believed that the control he had over the conditions of work of being a teacher was a key reason he was still at the job.

> I think as a teacher though, that is one of the best occupations that I could be in for the disease. If I had to do any other work, I fear that I probably wouldn't be able to sustain it and I would probably die away rather quickly. I have a great deal of control over the classes I work with and I am also a coordinator at the school. So I kind of look out for my own schedule and I have some perks. (bisexual black male)

Fatigue can affect mental as well as physical aspects of work, worsening memory loss or confusion. Chad had serious lapses in his ability to do the job.

> Like with the fatigue thing, I forgot how to use the cash register. I have been there for seven years. I got to the cash register and I had to ring

a bill in and I was almost in tears, because I forgot how to use the cash register. My mind just went blank and this has happened two times in the last year. I called a waitress and I said, "Marsha, this is Chad. You know me, I am so dizzy, well . . ." And then it came back to me. . . . Then the second time it happened, I waited ten minutes and it came back, I didn't call anyone. . . . Generally I don't feel tired, because I just turn my mind off to my body when I am working. I am a robot. (gay white male).

Similarly, Nick reported:

So I get tired during the day, and I'll get confused and . . . . and there are times when words come out backwards. You do think about it [dementia]. I used to have to do that [nap] and I don't any more . . . I think it was more psychological then. . . . because I had this disease and this is what I am supposed to do. (gay white male)

The best solution to fatigue is rest, an activity typically at odds with work. Some people found the leeway to get some rest on the job. Gordon informed his employer of his HIV status and asked to be allowed extra rest at work.

The key is going to be rest, getting plenty of rest. That is part of the battle. That is my priority. And they [employer] said fine. But it is still, we get a lot of part-time people coming in and a lot of times they think because there is no one in my office, they will open the door at 2:00 or 2:30 in the afternoon, and I am sitting there sleeping, and they never say anything. The part-time people, I am sure that they go back home, "This guy is probably making a zillion dollars, and I open the door and he is just sleeping in his room." (heterosexual white male)

While Gordon had the support of management and was therefore not worried about what people might think of his napping on the job, Clarence had not told his supervisor. He used the fact that his job required a great deal of travel in his car to take time for rest.

I need just a 20 minute nap somewhere, and I'll be out in a company car and I'll just find some place to park and just drop my head down and sleep, or on my way back down, I may stop at home, sometimes just ten minutes will do it. I just need a small time period, but basically I think I am doing OK. (gay aboriginal/white male)

Clarence resolved the conflicting demands of career and AIDS by "power napping," as he put it. He had determined to continue working as long as possible, and died less than a year later.

Two others tried to limit work-related stress in place of resting. As a teacher, Robbie had the room to pace his own activities.

It's made me concentrate more on doing things that do not build up a lot of stress. I avoid overtaxing myself with a lot of activity at one point. If I see for example the marks, the grades, are coming up soon, then I don't plan to do a lot of other things as well. . . . And I'm always very conscious of kids being ill, with colds and so on. (gay white male)

Daniel refused a promotion in order to avoid increased stress.

Right now I'm a night auditor at a motel and I was the assistant manager, you know, and maybe I should be the manager now and maybe because of the disease maybe that's why I haven't gotten that far yet because I'm worried to take on the extra pressure, responsibility. And what happens if I do get sick? (gay white male)

Workplace stress may be compounded by pressures mounting in other areas of life. Nick described the strains he faced because he was supporting an HIV-positive lover.

It is a strain and [I] feel it is continuing because he is positive. It is a tremendous pressure. I cannot miss work. If I don't feel well I go into work. Sometimes I am better off at work than being home, but I can't afford not to go to work, so I do. (gay white male)

Management may look upon washroom breaks with suspicion, seeing them as a violation of the requirements of work discipline. Yet diarrhea can leave the employee with little choice. Warren, a factory worker in his twenties, had to justify his washroom use.

I can do anything, everything that I could do before. They asked me about going to the bathroom so much and I gave them the medical paperwork, stating why I go. (gay black male)

Sick time and time for doctor's appointments pose similar problems. Crystal worked for an AIDS agency which was supportive of her need for time for doctor's appointments, but did not have adequate provisions for longer illness.

My boss understands all my doctor's appointments I have to keep. That is the part that I thought that wouldn't be understood, but she does. Only when I don't have the time to cover it, sick time, personal time, and then it is like if I get sick and don't get a check to cover my bills, by me working I cannot get any outside help, from any other agency. (heterosexual black female)

Personal appearance can play a role in job performance, both as a condition for meeting the public and as a determinant of one's own self-esteem and sense of competence. Chad decided this:

> I told her if I was ever to get sick and look sickly, I do not want to come to work and have everybody look at me looking ugly. I am very well kept. I am not going to go into work with lesions on my face. I freak out when I get a zit. . . . I am not going to go into work all ugly and bald, and big black circles under my eyes. (gay white male)

Finally, illness may increase the sense of personal vulnerability. Nick reported that seropositivity had made him more cautious at work.

> I don't create controversy. Before I used to. It is not a dramatic change, but I was always on the forefront of an issue. I no longer do that to the same extent. I will express myself, but I don't put myself in the forefront. I am not in the limelight, so I am being identified as being out there, existing, but not being part of the woodwork either. I have gotten away from that. I want to take the middle of the road approach, like half the other people out there. It is a lot easier. Go with the flow. I have had to. (gay white male)

Coping with HIV-infection on the job raises a range of serious issues. Many become especially concerned about maintaining their employment in order to maintain their health benefits at the same time as they have to deal with symptoms that may compromise their work performance. Yet, even people who perform well may be perceived by employers as not doing so if they violate the norms of work-discipline through resting, frequent bathroom visits, or time off for doctor's appointments.[3]

Telling Co-Workers

While co-workers can act as a source of support, many are poorly informed about AIDS and have fears generally not connected to any actual risk of transmission in the workplace (Lamm and Brewer 1990:737). Vernon withdrew from social contact with co-workers after being diagnosed.

> No one does know. They sense there is a change in me. I'm, my social level is like zero. I go into work, I don't talk to anybody, I don't even say good morning to anybody but that is just part of my depression about where I am at. (gay white male)

The research on AIDS phobia shows clearly that homophobia is its primary determinant (Nelkin 1987; Triplet and Sugarman 1987). Jeff reported that AIDS phobic attitudes existed even among health care workers.

One day on the floor where we were discussing this whole issue of AIDS
and homosexuality and that kind of thing, one person said, they
should all be isolated in a commune or shot. Now this is a nurse I
worked with for a year and a half, shoulder to shoulder. . . . Now I'm
sitting there going, "Now Sally, how could you? You know I'm gay. You
know I'm not a child molester. This is a terribly homophobic attitude
coming out of you, this whole lack of information as another professional about the issue of AIDS." . . . It was just astounding. (gay
white/aboriginal male)

Wayne found co-workers quick to use AIDS as a weapon of homophobic
harassment even though they knew nothing of his sero-status.

I heard they caught wind that I was gay. I had a pop or coffee sitting
there. "Don't forget that he has AIDS." [These were co-workers?] Yeah,
they know that I am strong enough where I'll, they could be sued for
slander. I ignore it. . . . So I try to teach them or try to let them know.
(gay white male)

Peter's supportive employer recommended that he not tell co-workers of
his seropositivity.

He did tell me, however, that the only thing that he would ask is that I
could stay on as long as I wanted as long as I did not let the rest of the
employees know. . . . We had only, like, nine employees but I mean we
had these redneck guys . . . that were repairmen. (gay white male)

The barriers of silence that surround AIDS and HIV can make it difficult
to sustain relationships with co-workers. Gordon informed his co-workers of his HIV-status at a meeting and found them supportive. Indeed, at
times, he found them irritatingly solicitous.

It was just basically concern about how-are-you-feeling type of stuff.
That I hear much more often then I ever did before, I hear that everyday. "Are you losing weight? Is that, has it got anything to do with HIV?"
It is irritating, but I just can't find a way around it. Once you go public, you can't say I am only this much public. Once you have stated it,
people say it hurts their feelings. They feel that they are really concerned. They don't understand that you have been asked that question ten times already and the eleventh one you are going to bark at.
(heterosexual white male)

Tom agonized over how to inform co-workers of the reason he was leaving on a disability pension and eventually struck on a creative solution.
With the assistance of his supervisor, he sent personal letters to employees at their homes to explain his departure.

That provided an opportunity for them to have an idea of feeling and thinking about this on their own apart from a desk drop, where there would be an opinion within hearing range, where one person invents it, and then the other people embrace it, because it is convenient . . . and my experience has been that that has been a very positive experience. The responses were such that, I received probably over 100 cards and letters. (gay white male).

The individualized response of personal letters undercut the tendency for workplace gossip and instant opinion formation. His honesty and self-revelation elicited an outpouring of sympathy and a "send off" which he found to be both touching and affirming.

Workplace AIDS Policies

An official policy on AIDS should ease much of the insecurity of HIV-positive people at work and assuage the fears and prejudices of co-workers and management. Bill Patterson (1989:40) notes that fewer than ten percent of American companies have AIDS policies, and few are evident among the employers of participants in this study. Even where they exist, people living with HIV do not necessarily trust that they will be followed. Frank works in a hospital with a policy on AIDS but he had little confidence that his co-workers had been adequately educated on the subject.

They should be but they are not. They are very unprepared. They have an AIDS policy, but it surely isn't followed to a great degree. (gay white male)

Robbie, who is a teacher, felt that his colleagues would not be prepared to deal with a case of AIDS in their immediate environs. Further, he was worried that ways would be found within the official policies to remove him from work.

I couldn't even predict. All of them have been trained in this and so on, but I don't think it's sunk in that it could be so close to them. Well, as far as discrimination or anything like that, that's definitely out. . . . I've never read a policy, but they can't fire me. I would still be in my job and so on, but I think there would be pressure put on to put me on long term disability or something just to cover up any kind of social implications. (gay white male)

Tom described a policy that was implemented through educational broadcasts in the workplace which he attended with his superior.

I went with my supervisor, she knowing that I was gay. She has known that for years. We are close friends. I went with her to a company sponsored broadcast that went to all the plants, say three years ago maybe, about the AIDS question. That from the union and management got together with a panel of doctors and they satellited it to every plant location and anyone who was interested could watch it. It basically said no risk using the washrooms, cafeterias, and company commitment in this area. (gay white male)

In this situation, where the employee knows the company AIDS policy, and knows that the supervisor knows, a policy is likely to feel more like a source of support. Jim assumed that such policies are the province of large firms rather than smaller businesses or agencies.

It is actually something that I haven't thought about. I thought if I was in a large enough corporation, say for example, I was to get into General Motors, that would be something I might think about myself. To kind of research it, try to find out. No, because I think that is a big enough corporation with all its entities, that it might be a need for that. But where I work at now, with a local social service agency . . . I don't think it is a large enough work staff. (bisexual black male)

While some very large firms, particularly those with trade unions, have developed specific AIDS policies that provide some assurance for employees living with HIV, small firms can sometimes meet their needs because of their emphasis on personal relations. Philip worked in a firm run by his family.

Being in a family business, it is quite flexible. . . . We are a very, very small company. Basically we have no policies. . . . All I know is my dad said at the time, when I told them, he said, "You can have whatever time you take off, you take it, whether you are there or not your check will always be there." (gay white male)

Dale Masi (1990:42) identifies the ideal AIDS policy as including four aspects: specific education about HIV transmission at work, an approach that treats AIDS like other chronic illnesses, a commitment to supporting people with HIV as long as possible in their jobs, and general AIDS education. Nick was aware of only the first of these areas being covered in the policy at the laboratory where he worked.

The only policy that I am aware of, since we work with blood specimens, and we work with sputum and various other body fluids, the only policy I know covers the universal precautions in handling of specimens. . . . But that is the policy of [a] work-induced positive test as opposed to somebody from the outside. So I know of no policy that covers that. (gay white male)

AIDS service organizations might be expected to be model employers in terms of workplace policies but even their practices may not attain Masi's ideal. Whether due to limited funds, an inability to obtain appropriate benefits packages, or a failure to prioritize policies to safeguard employ- ees with HIV. Rick reported that his workplace was not fully prepared with policies covering the conditions of HIV-positive employees.

> We need to make it more clear as far as the policies of this organiza- tion. There is nothing in place . . . for any life-threatening illness or ter- minal illness. (heterosexual white male)

In work sites without a full educational component, it may fall to sero- positive workers to try to enlighten those around them. This could be particularly difficult for those who fear exposing themselves through their interest and knowledge of AIDS. Jeff remarked,

> I did reasonably well at educating my work peers in relation to the issues but never to the risk of revealing to a lot of them that what they're talking about for me is what I'm living right now. (gay white/aboriginal male)

Frank, a hospital worker, had to attempt both general education to chal- lenge irrational fears and specific instruction about workplace precau- tions, all without exposing his own HIV-status.

> I have got very disgusted with people at work. . . . The head of our department is very AIDS phobic. I did bring him information to try and educate him somewhat about AIDS but I presented to him as com- ing from somebody who was not HIV positive, someone who just told him he was AIDS phobic, one person to another. . . . I have to take [responsibility] sometimes, just regular blood precautions at work, as far as even trying to remind people that they have a bad habit of not wearing gloves when they should. (gay white male)

On the other hand, Gordon who had publicly disclosed his seropositiv- ity at work found himself overwhelmed with requests for information.

> I started getting a whole bunch of calls last summer, and 200 explana- tions. It is not fun. It doesn't stress me, other than I want to go home. I get a phone call from somebody at 4:45, and a guy says, "Gord, I just found out you are dealing with this HIV, hemophilia thing. What is it

all about?" and I spend two hours on the phone and they feel better.
So I am doing it. I am doing something very useful, and it helps me a
lot. Gee it is very tiring. That is one of the things, that is the only negative I can say, I have to give the same story 200 times. (heterosexual
white male)

Leaving Employment

People living with HIV also leave their jobs for reasons other than the
fear of discriminatory measures. Shifting priorities as well as changes in
physical, mental, and emotional condition may lead to ending employment. Two people we interviewed left their jobs immediately after being
tested. Ray quit his job directly after getting his test results.

> I went right to work and quit, and told him, told the owner of the
> restaurant. . . . no notice or anything, but he knew there was some-
> thing up too, because he knew I had a doctor's appointment. His
> daughter told him. So he was actually very good. And that is basically
> it. I sort of hid out for a while. (gay white male)

A positive test result can suddenly make the world look quite different,
leading to a reassessment of priorities, including the place of work in
one's life. Jeff regretted his decision to sharply reorient his priorities
soon after testing positive.

> I resigned my position. This is the one foolish thing financially I think
> I did for myself. I resigned my position with the federal government
> before my AIDS diagnosis while I was still in that seropositive state
> thinking I was going to go back to school and get myself re-educated
> and move into another field and I would probably get into another as-
> secure disability pension plan. (gay white/aboriginal male)

The security promised by benefits plans may seem much more significant later in the syndrome than in an earlier asymptomatic period. Many
people with HIV are relatively young and may share with their peers a
lack of anticipation of pension issues. At the same time, HIV infection
can generate new needs that can be met only through changing jobs or
withdrawing from paid employment. Alex, who had worked in a facility
for teenagers, left his job both to be near home in case of HIV-related illness and to stop wearing himself out with physically demanding work.

> I left because time was passing on, so I better get on back home. In
> case something did happen I would be here. . . . Running down the
> hall, breaking up fights, stuff like that. I figured I was getting too old

for that, so I said, "Let me leave, now, so I won't tire myself too much."
(bisexual black male)

Jason left his job and described it as "retirement," reflecting the decision of some HIV infected people to withdraw from the strain of paid
employment.

> I retired. I was in a space where . . . I was making it to work and get-
> ting home and I would be so tired that I had to go to bed before I
> could go eat. And there just had to be more to life than . . . [working
> as] a payroll clerk. . . . They were going to kill me if I let them. (gay
> white male)

HIV infection itself can be a source of stress that makes it difficult to sustain paid employment. Todd said,

> I couldn't work because of the psychological part, you know. I lost con-
> fidence in looking for the jobs, thinking it's a death sentence, what's
> the point of working? . . . . That was probably all through bad judgment
> and reaction and desperation, you know, that that had happened. (gay
> white male).

The "psychological part" may include, in varying proportions, depression or fatigue, which in turn, can contribute to difficulty in concentrat-
ing or remembering. Bob left work in response to these problems.

> I tried working, after getting out of hospital, seven months. I just
> couldn't handle it, couldn't look at a computer screen any more,
> couldn't remember things. (gay white male).

These stresses may be compounded by the illness or death of friends,
lovers, and other members of social networks. Nichols describes this condition as "bereavement overload," a condition exacerbated by the fact
that "the stigma associated with AIDS forces those people to cope with AIDS
privately, secretively and at a distance" (Tedlow and Marram 1991:21).
Roger found these dilemmas to be debilitating.

> I worked for a little while, a couple days a week, from December right
> up until Elliot passed away. I was trying to do this job. I couldn't.
> December, January, February and March, I was too sick, and I was psy-
> chologically just a wreck, so I ended up losing the job and I really
> haven't worked since. (gay white male)

Some people leave work for job-specific reasons. Ninia left the sex trade
as she felt she could no longer continue with it.

I had to quit my career, the one thing I knew I could do, and I am scared to get a job. (heterosexual white female)

In the United States some HIV-infected people had to leave their jobs to "spend down" their assets in order to gain eligibility for medical coverage. U.S. public medical care programs generally cover only people with limited income and assets, or senior citizens. Workplace plans generally cover only conditions that develop after the person is employed in a certain workplace and often include sizeable co-payments (discussed further in Chapter 7).

Losing a Job

The majority of respondents were not currently employed. Many had either lost or left jobs after they were diagnosed. Those who continue to work often fear the possibility of job loss, due either to discrimination or a decline in their own ability to do the job. While some people reach moments in which they are unable to continue their employment, job loss is often not a result of strict medical necessity. Five of the participants in this study mentioned being fired because of employers' overtly discriminatory practices and others left jobs in anticipation of such problems. These findings are similar to those reported by Rose Weitz (1990:31; 1991:123–25).

Despite being contrary to legislation in both Ontario and Michigan, many of those who were dismissed did not pursue possible legal redress. At a time when they were coping financial losses, health problems, and a range of other difficulties detailed in these chapters, many found the prospect of legal action to be an additional burden that would be too expensive and too stressful.

Andy was fired after disclosing his HIV status to his supervisor. He was appealing his dismissal through a union procedure.

I had been stupid enough to tell my supervisor that I was HIV positive and that was why I was so tired. They turned around and fired me over it. They didn't say that was what it was. They never will. They came out with a bad evaluation. Went for the sack in August and I've got a grievance pending now that's due to be heard. (gay white male)

He believed that the dismissal was connected to a sharp increase in insurance costs facing his employers.

They were scared. They were going to end up with catastrophic health care costs. They had gotten their premiums for their insurance. . . .

tripled in that three month stretch before I was fired, so they had to
change carriers again and they were scared to death of catastrophic
health care costs. So they'd have rather dumped me that be stuck with
a huge health care bill.

The U.S. medical system provides incentives for employers and insurance companies to rid themselves of potentially costly claims. This poses
grave hardships to people who are forced out of medical plans at the
very moment they need them most (see Gostin 1993).

Brad, a private duty nurse, was fired despite a frank discussion with his
employer about precautions.

> I had to tell my boss during the time I was hospitalized. After three
> days, four days, he wanted to know why I was away . . . in that hospital,
> and he said, "Brad, it's AIDS isn't it?" Prior to that we had a big discus-
> sion. . . . He said, "Brad, if you were ever HIV positive, obviously I don't
> think I would want you working for me." I was doing private duty nurs-
> ing for him and I did quite a bit. As far as bowel stimulation, bathing,
> that type of thing, he was just real nervous about it. And I tried to
> explain, "Well I wear rubber gloves when I do the bowel stimulation
> anyway. What's the big deal?" But he was still very uncomfortable with
> that. (gay white male)

Lacking a union, he was fired without benefits and given a very small
cash settlement.

> There was $1,200 in cash. He said, "That will help you get home," which
> it did . . . $1,200 was measly compared to the two months I sat there and
> spent what I had in the bank and had no money. (gay white male).

Devon quit his job after hospitalization. He felt his employers knew the
nature of his illness and that consequences would follow. He was then
fired from the next job he took.

> They knew I was in isolation. They put two and two together. There was
> one person there, I thought that they knew what was going on, so I left
> that job, and went to . . . this other job only to get fired because they
> found out. (gay black male)

An HIV diagnosis soon raises an employee's sexual orientation in his
employer's mind. Where gay people have no legal protection from discrimination, their continued employment may then depend entirely
on the prejudices of management.[4] David found that his partner's illness exposed his sexuality to his employer. He was fired on the day his
lover died.

But when he died, they fired me at my job, my day job, and so I was left without, I didn't have a job . . . I had asked for a leave, when I brought him home from the hospital to die, and they had agreed to give it to me. I never disclosed to them. If they asked me, I would have told them, but I never officially said Lenny has AIDS and I never officially said to them I am gay. It was a very conservative office. I am sure they had figured it all out, and the one partner was going to give me the leave and then three days later they called. Lenny had died that morning. I came home to a message on the phone that the job was gone. (gay white male)

After being fired, he tried to resume the sales-related job which he had left for a steadier income during his partner's illness. His employer, however, would not rehire him.

She sat down and said that she really hated to be like the other people. That was just breaking her heart. She just hated to do that to me, but she worked so hard to build that up, and that there were too many people in the office that knew about me and knew about Lenny and she was afraid that the business would go down the tubes, so it would probably be better if I didn't come back to work. That was two [jobs], so that devastated me more than anything really as far as knocking the props out from under me. (gay white male)

Some people resign in anticipation of HIV-related discrimination. The situation of Ted, a teacher, was particularly revealing. He faced growing anxiety as the knowledge of his HIV-status seemed to move closer to his workplace. The pressure of maintaining secrecy in a potentially hostile environment was immense. The problems seemed to be getting too close when one of his former students was hired by his doctor.

She had access to the records and probably came upon my name, doing the demographics work that she was assigned to do. She was a former graduate of this high school and knew that I worked here. There are also other kinds of inconsistencies too. Like a parent. I'd had trouble with a student, phoned to see the parents, and he ended up being the vice president of finance at the [hospital] where my records were. It got too close, so when I resigned I did so almost in relief (gay white male).

Lacking any sense of job security as a gay man and as a seropositive person, he preferred to protect himself from consequences he saw as all too imminent.

The remedial measures available for cases of unfair dismissal or similar situations of discrimination often do not meet the needs of people living with HIV. The major remedy that respondents mention is legal action, though this usually comes up in the context of explaining why they would not pursue such actions. David explained that he would not pursue legal action after his AIDS-related dismissal.

> I don't earn a lot of money, but I don't spend a lot of money. And there isn't anything I have a real burning desire to do, that I can't or don't do. And it takes a lot of energy to get angry and to hate someone and to do those kinds of things so it is just not worth the effort to pursue it. (gay white male)

The pursuit of a law suit requires time and money. Even Devon, who felt he had a solid case, did not pursue it because "I didn't have the energy."

Unions should be able to provide an alternate avenue of recourse. Andy was fired for HIV-related causes but specifically requested that the union not use that information in the grievance process.

> The union, I told them what the actual thing was but I told them I don't want to file a grievance on those grounds. (gay white male)

Few of the people we interviewed were in unionized workplaces, reflecting the job sectors in which the respondents were located as well as the relative weakness of the union movement in the United States.[5] Not only are nonunionized workers extremely vulnerable to summary action but they also have less access to benefits packages (discussed further in the next chapter).

AIDS and HIV raise a number of issues around work discipline, job loss, relations among workers, discrimination, and health and safety that unions could address. Evan, who had a partner suffering from AIDS, pressed the reluctant leadership of his union to take a stand.

> One of the people who is a specialist in health care policy . . . for the [union], said we should not introduce a resolution on AIDS and AIDS testing at this [union] meeting because the rank and file would stand up—given their ignorance and fear—would stand up and might well vote it down. . . . I said, "That's outrageous." I said, "By the time you guys make up your minds . . . about what you want to do about this, there will be more people who will have died of this than died in the Vietnam war." (gay white male)

Even among union members, the participants in this study seldom mentioned turning to their unions for redress, indicating that unions were either absent or ineffective in creating situations where workers could approach them in times of trouble and feel safe in assuming that they would receive protection. Yet contract provisions that protect people living with HIV would also serve many others in the workplace by allowing working parents, pregnant women, or people with other illnesses the flexibility appropriate to their needs.[6]

Joblessness

Paid employment can provide a place in the world. The loss of a job can trigger feelings of displacement, uselessness, and dependency. Anne Ritter (1989:36) writes, "People fail to realize how much work impacts their lives until they stop. Work is a diversion—it is social and constructive." Devon described the shift out of paid employment as a turning point in the trajectory of the syndrome for him.

> After I was fired, that is when my health really took a turn for the worse, the symptoms they just seemed to get worse and worse. (gay black male)

Joblessness can also effect the dynamics of domestic relationships as financial contribution to the household figures among the symbolic exchanges between couples. Ninia reported that her job status became an issue in disagreements with her husband.

> Sometimes we argue. "You need me. I am paying the rent." It is not [nice], but he throws it in my face and we argue. So it is giving him a big macho feeling. (heterosexual white female).

Two men described their current job status as "housewife," an ironic reference to the identification of domestic labor as "women's work." Still, gay men may experience a different relationship to domestic labor in comparison with their heterosexual counterparts because their domestic arrangements do not duplicate the traditional household division of labor. Lesbians and gay men have often been innovators in breaking into gender-defined work both in the domestic and wage-labor economies. Wayne used the "housewife" designation in a possibly self-deprecating manner in responding to a question about how he spent his time:

> Sending out resumes and going to interviews. Nothing really, watch TV in the house, make sure Ian has clean clothes. Little housewife, I guess. (gay white male)

Peter, however, seemed to be using the "housewife" category to establish a way of valuing his new life.

I keep very busy. I go to support groups twice a week. I have breakfast with a friend two or three times a week. . . . I do all the laundry, all the cooking, all the cleaning, and most of the yard work for a very large home [a household of four adults]. . . . I'm a housewife and I'm every bit as busy as a housewife with a couple of kids. (gay white male)

Previously employed people with HIV may find themselves with plenty of time on their hands, good health, and a sense that their life is in suspension. Fred was proud of his previous work and found his current daily regime dull:

Definitely bored. If it wasn't for thinking about getting my apartment together, I would be totally bored. I think I am into television too much. I think I am into soap operas too much. Given any day of the week, I could tell you what is on TV from 12:30 in the afternoon up until 6:30 the next morning . . . I think I am wasting my mind actually. (gay black male)

New endeavors can provide a renewed sense of direction and worth. Volunteer work filled the place that work had once occupied in Peter's life.

Volunteering was really not for them but for me. And I told them point blank, I said, "I'm not here to help them, I'm here to help me." . . . And I strongly recommend it. (gay white male)

Not everyone is disturbed by having time on their hands. Lemuel described the benefits of relaxation.

We feel like we got to be doing something. I learned how to relax a long time ago: read, look at television, I don't feel guilt about it, look at old movies on television. I don't always have the energy or the desire to get and run to the support group or what have you. So spend time? Let's say that time spends me. (gay black male)

Conclusion

The workplace poses a number of problems for people with HIV infection. Not least among these problems is blatant AIDS phobic discrimination where some employers show no hesitation in terminating the livelihood of individuals in the hour of their greatest need. Legal remedies to discrimination based on disability often prove to be cumbersome, expensive, and inaccessible, while unions reach few workers and frequently lack effective methods of redress. Still fewer jurisdictions offer even the possibility of legal recourse to the anti-gay discrimination which accompanies an HIV diagnosis. HIV disease at times also raises physical and mental problems in getting work done, requiring employers to provide some flexibility to the worker. In some cases, especially in large corporations with explicit AIDS policies, in small businesses with well-established personal relationships, and in workplaces with gay co-workers or managers, HIV-positive workers find the support necessary to help meet the challenges of chronic illness. In a few cases, especially among former drug users, testing HIV-positive is the occasion for reorganizing one's life and reentering the job market. More frequently, HIV-positive workers in jurisdictions without universal health insurance face the prospect of having to fall into penury in order to acquire medical services. The binational nature of this sample allows us to examine how two very different systems of medical service impact on the experience on HIV disease, explored further in the next chapter.

Chapter Seven

EXPERIENCING HEALTH CARE
IN TWO NATIONS

From the earliest interviews it became clear that there was one major recurring difference in the experience of life with HIV in Canada and the United States. Canadians take access to health care largely for granted while many Americans face substantial obstacles to obtaining the services they require. We did not emphasize American-Canadian comparisons in previous chapters as national differences did not emerge as an issue relevant in other areas of life. In general terms, there is a great deal of similarity in the experience of living with HIV on both sides of the United States-Canada border. As well, the qualitative methods we employed provide the basis for only cautious generalizations about these differences as we did not sample or analyze data in ways that might provide a systematic basis for a comparative discussion.

A binational comparison is complicated by the fact that study participants in the two countries differed in several ways apart from their place of residence. Among the U.S. participants, there was a much higher representation of women, people of color, drug users, and men who have sex with men but do not identify as gay. These demographic differences stem from the different epidemiological pattern of HIV disease in the two countries. The large increase in the rate of HIV infection among the urban poor in the United States has, so far, no parallel in Canada. Merrill Singer (1994:933) argues that the spread of AIDS in the inner cities of the United States is just one feature of "an explosive chain-reaction of interconnected epidemics." This demographic profile likely heightens the contrasts between the two health care systems as middle class people in the United States are more likely to have comprehensive health insurance and thus resemble Canadians in their access to health services.

Public vs Private Health Care

This binational sample of people living with HIV permits a comparison of the ways in which the organization of health care on a national scale affects the experiences of people dealing with a life-threatening syndrome. Intense public debates over the relative merits of public and private health care systems have been occurring in both the United States and Canada in recent years. While many conflicting interest groups have advanced claims about the economics, availability, and effectiveness of each system, the experience of patients has typically received little attention.

Health care coverage in Canada is universal, relatively comprehensive, and has no user payment (or copayment) for basic health services. Provincial governments administer health insurance within parameters set by the federal government, which also covers some of the costs. In Ontario, medical service users pay no direct premiums for health care coverage. A combination of federal and provincial taxes cover costs, including a payroll tax levied on employers specifically to cover health. The provincial government compensates physicians or other service providers, who are not allowed to charge any fees additional to those received from the government on a fee-for-service basis.

The comprehensiveness of the Canadian system is bounded by a series of noteworthy exclusions. Dental care is not covered. Many crucial treatments, such as medications or corrective lenses, are not included unless covered through supplementary benefits provided through employment or through specific social assistance programs. None of these characteristics of the Canadian system are historically guaranteed or fixed. With health care taking a substantial portion of government budgets at a time when deficit reduction has become a leading priority, the attempt to reduce costs has brought the entire system under review. Nevertheless, the social democratic government of Ontario introduced an extension of coverage (shortly after the completion of interviews reflected in this study), in order to pay for the drug costs of people with "catastrophic" illnesses including AIDS. At the same time, cost cutting has raised the possibility of the contraction of the current system of easy access.

Overall, study participants living in Canada take their access to health care for granted, with the notable exception of payment for medication. Not surprisingly, access to health care does not emerge as an important issue for them. In contrast, U.S. respondents spend considerable time and energy in attempting to gain access to medical services. The United States is the only major industrialized country without a national health system providing universal and relatively comprehensive access to medical services (Navarro 1992:vii),[1] relying instead on health insurance plans provided by the corporate sector. This private, profit-oriented medical system is the most expensive in the world, measured as a percentage of the Gross Domestic Product or on a per capita basis (Organization for Economic Cooperation and Development 1992:18). Despite its cost, significant numbers of people totally lack health insurance coverage.

Employment-related health insurance plays the key role in the U.S. system. In the words of the Organization for Economic Cooperation and Development (1992:38) report, "In view of the importance of employer-based insurance, it is not surprising that those having only weak connection to the labor market have a high probability of being uninsured." Further, many people who are employed are not insured through their workplace. Only some workplaces offer medical insurance as a benefit. Even where this benefit is available, some individuals are disqualified on the basis of a "pre-existing condition," that is, an illness that preceded employment at that workplace.[2] Thomas Bodenheimer (1992:275) estimates that 81 million Americans have medical problems that might be considered to be "pre-existing conditions." Peter Franks, Carolyn Clancy and Marthe Gold (1993:737) state that the number of people without medical insurance in the United States increased through the 1980s and reached 35.4 million in 1991. Adults and children who are not insured are less likely to seek or receive medical attention or treatment (Spillman 1992:462). As a result, uninsured people have a higher mortality rate, even if factors such as employment, education, age, and income are taken into account (Franks, Clancy and Gold 1993:739–40). Moreover, many of those who are insured have less than full coverage. Bodenheimer (1992:274–75) reports that an additional 20 million people are underinsured, meaning that they would not be adequately covered in the event of a serious illness. He points out that 75 percent of plans include user payments (or copayments) of at least 20 percent. These user payments can be a major obstacle to seeking out regular medical services or expensive procedures.

People living with HIV infection are particularly likely to be excluded from private insurance. Profit-oriented insurance companies have strong incentives for excluding individuals with potentially expensive conditions. Risk pooling confronts employers, particularly in small workplaces, with the threat of dramatically increased premiums to cover even one individual with a condition requiring expensive treatment. As Daniel Fife and James McAnaney (1993:516) write, "Private medical insurance is increasingly failing to meet the need for funding AIDS care."[3]

Job loss is the primary reason that people with HIV lose private insurance coverage (Kass, et al. 1991:253–54). People who lose their job have the option under federal legislation of continuing coverage (which runs out after 18 months) by paying the premium themselves, though this is often prohibitively expensive (Kass et al. 1991:253). Those who are employed can also find themselves uninsured if their HIV infection is classified as a pre-existing condition. Even if they are not excluded from benefits on this basis, they may find themselves quite suddenly cut off when their HIV status is identified. Courts have upheld employers who switch from insurance plans that cover HIV and AIDS to plans that do not (Gostin 1993). Other plans cap benefits (or set a lifetime maximum) for people with HIV-related claims, raise premiums to unaffordable heights once HIV-related claims are made, or avoid insuring people perceived as being at higher risk on the basis of occupation, sexual orientation, or an HIV-antibody test (Fife and McAnaney 1993:516).

Overall, then, people living with HIV face a number of obstacles that may prevent them from being covered by private insurance. Those with lower incomes and a more marginal relationship to the labor market are unlikely to have private insurance coverage in the first place while those who are better off may lose coverage because of the termination of employment or provisions excluding them from plans, as discussed above. In a study by John Fleshman and Vincent Mor (1993:183), 17 percent of participants had lost private insurance coverage since testing HIV-positive. As a result, government-run programs like Medicaid play a crucial role in the health care coverage of people living with HIV. Indeed, more people living with HIV move from private insurance to Medicaid than do those with other illnesses (Kass et al. 1991:254). The role of Medicaid in the funding of HIV care has increased through the history of the AIDS epidemic (Green and Arno 1990, Fife and McAnaney 1993). This is, in part, due to the demographic shift in the patterns of

HIV infection in the United States, where the urban poor make up an increasing proportion of the HIV-positive population. It cannot, however, be explained in these terms alone. People with HIV are increasingly reliant on Medicaid funding even accounting for these demographic factors (Fife and McAnaney 1993:514, Fleshman and Mor 1993:186, Green and Arno 1990:1263–64).

Medicaid and other government-funded plans do not automatically rescue people who are not covered by private insurance. People are included in these plans only if they meet specific criteria. Low-income women and children, particularly in single parent families, may qualify through the Aid to Families with Dependent Children (AFDC) program (Ellwood, Fanning and Dodds 1991:1037). They generally qualify for this coverage even if they are not HIV-positive. Others must be classified as disabled and have incomes or assets below government-established poverty lines. Those whose incomes and assets are not already below these poverty lines may qualify for Medicaid when they have lost or "spent down" their assets and savings to the point where they meet poverty criteria because their medical bills exceed their income (McCormack 1990:57). Many people living with HIV obtain coverage through this route.[4]

Medicaid provides a fairly full range of services to people living with AIDS. However, it does not necessarily provide for the outpatient care required for the treatment of HIV as a chronic illness (Green and Arno 1990:1265). Indeed, people who qualify for Medicaid through spending down their assets are unlikely to be covered unless they are already quite ill. These medically needy enrollees tend to be covered by Medicaid only for the final stages of their illness (Ellwood et al. 1991:1044).

People who do not qualify for Medicaid may meet the criteria for some state or locally funded programs that provide medical services to those on General Assistance, a social welfare program for the indigent (which was abolished by a new Republican governor of Michigan shortly after the completion of interviews for this study). Two of the participants in this study reported that they received this kind of assistance (called County Care in our study area). As will be discussed below, they said that Medicaid provided a much fuller range of services.

There are many holes in the American private insurance system through which people with HIV may fall. People with low incomes are likely to have never been covered. Others may lose their coverage due to job loss or exclusion by insurance providers. Even those who are covered may be underinsured. The Medicaid net will catch some of those who fall through the holes, but only if they meet disability and poverty criteria. In contrast, the Canadian system provides universal and relatively comprehensive coverage. It is not surprising, then, that participants in this study living in the United States discussed health care coverage a great deal while it did not emerge as an issue in the Canadian interviews. Indeed, Lemuel stated that organizing medical coverage was a top priority for people living with HIV/AIDS.

> So that is the most important thing to me, get your medical together, your medical, your insurance. (gay black male)

Access to health care is important for the physical health of people living with HIV, but also for the overall sense of well-being. Concern about access to health care creates very real stress for people living with HIV in the United States. Vernon was worried both about being cut off insurance when he needed it most and about the exposure of his HIV status at work through insurance issues.

> Now I don't know how . . . the insurance company and my employer are going to react once they realize I start getting medication for [being] HIV positive. I worry, I am fearful, that perhaps the insurance agent that got the company signed up for this policy may come back to the boss, knowing that it is a small company, and he can just freely call the boss and say, "One of your employees is taking AZT. You know what that stuff costs? You know what that is for?" (U.S. white gay male)

David was concerned that he could lose his benefits just when he most needed them.

> And you take those benefits for granted but once you are faced with a very serious illness, and suddenly simply because you have lost that job, that goes with it. It is a very significant thing (U.S. gay white male).

Qualifying for Health Coverage in the United States

Among the participants in this study living in the United States, three groups have good access to health care: those on Medicaid, those who receive Veteran's benefits, and family members of workers with a good workplace insurance program. Seventeen (36%) of the participants living in the United States mentioned that they are on Medicaid and three more are involved in the application process (which can be very lengthy).[5] Participants who have Medicaid coverage are generally satisfied with their access to health services. Rhonda was content with the scope of her health care coverage provided by the combination

of Medicaid and the assistance of an AIDS case management and refer-
ral agency.

> I am covered perfectly for everything. I have Medicaid. . . . Anything
> comes up the Medicaid doesn't cover, the AIDS Care Connection also
> helps you with that. (U.S. heterosexual black female)

Medicaid stands out among health care plans due to the absence of
copayments. People on Medicaid also have access to a greater range of
services than those on some other plans. Although Medicaid offers a
desirable health care plan, it comes at a cost. Lemuel mentioned the
impoverishment required for some recipients.

> Some people have to come down to get good medical insurance.
> Medicaid is about the best going at the moment. There is no copay-
> ment and then you have the option to go to wherever you want to,
> mostly wherever you want to go. (U.S. gay black male)

HIV-positive children receive coverage through Medicaid or other programs aimed at children with disabilities. Both Paula and Marcia were
satisfied that their children were properly covered for medical eventual-
ities through "crippled children's benefits."

The other government program that offers some Americans health
benefits equivalent to coverage at the Canadian level is assistance for war
veterans. This offers relatively comprehensive coverage without copayments, though treatment must be through Veterans Administration (VA)
facilities. Peter was satisfied with the extent of coverage he received.

> As it was, I ended up in the veterans' facility out in Ann Arbor and the
> treatment has been wonderful. The doctors have been great. . . . The VA
> . . . buys my prescriptions, takes care of my hospital, takes care of my out-
> patient. The only thing is I have to go there. . . . but everything is free.
> . . . The social worker there is great. . . . Anything you need they take
> care of. . . . You have to be discharged honorably from military service
> which I was back in 1971. . . . They cover all the medical, the psycholo-
> gist, the psychiatrist I have gone to for a year to get my head together.
> . . . Plus they even give me a pension to live on. (U.S. gay white male)

The U.S. military policy of overt discrimination against homosexual
men, both by refusing them admission and by expelling them through
dishonorable discharges, excludes a great many HIV-positive people
from this avenue of access to health care.

Other Americans who have quite comprehensive health care coverage are family members of employees with a benefits plan. Unionized

workplaces are particularly likely to have such plans; many others do not. Ninia is married to an autoworker from a unionized plant. Their coverage is quite complete, though it does include some copayments.

> We have Blue Cross. [My husband] works at GM, so we got real good coverage. Our office visits are like $20 each time, so we are real fortunate there. (U.S. heterosexual white female)

Although Gordon was covered by this kind of comprehensive package, he was concerned that his union might negotiate away parts of the plan given employer pressure to concede costly benefits.

> When the economy gets rocky, everybody starts looking at the cost and the cost of health insurance that your employer picks up is going up and up and up. It is the only thing that keeps skyrocketing here in the States. And it is really rough for a lot of companies to maintain full coverage. A lot of small companies have switched over to other policies which don't offer as much. (U.S. heterosexual white male)

Because of the failure of either union contracts or government legislation to recognize the family relationships of lesbians and gay men, none of the gay men in this study was able to include his partner in his family benefits.[6]

Apart from these three types of health plans, which cover a minority of the participants in this study, people living with HIV in the United States are left to search out health care as best they can.

The Struggle to Obtain Health Care

The United States health care system creates a number of access problems for people living with HIV. U.S. residents who are uninsured are personally responsible for their medical bills. Those who insure themselves may face onerous premiums. Even people with quite good coverage often end up stretching their finances to afford copayments. Some plans narrowly restrict the choice of doctors and treatments. Uninsured people are put in a position where they must avoid or minimize medical care. Some are employed in workplaces that do not have health care plans or are excluded from the plans that are offered. Others are unemployed and not eligible for Medicaid. People living with HIV who do not have insurance face enormous obstacles to managing their own health. Jordan could not find a job that provided health insurance.

> I haven't been able to get a job with medical insurance since I have been working. Since '83. (U.S. bisexual black male)

Some employers offer health care coverage to full time employees but not to part-timers or casual workers. Frank was not considered a full-time employee despite working almost forty hours a week.

> I am not full-time, even though I work 39 hours. So that is one way of getting around it, until you become a permanent full-time employee, then they would have to grant you insurance. There are ways of getting around it. (U.S. gay white male)

Sometimes people living with HIV remain uninsured even where workplace coverage is offered. Many health plans exclude people with pre-existing conditions or medical problems that predate employment at a particular workplace. Four of the participants in this research lost coverage when their HIV-status was defined as a pre-existing condition. Matt was cut off coverage at work when the insurance company defined his seropositivity as a pre-existing condition. He suddenly faced large medical bills from hospitals.

> They were real good until they decided it was a preexisting condition and wouldn't cover anymore. . . . The hospitals aren't going after the insurance companies, they are coming after me. (U.S. gay white male)

The insurance company cut Brad off coverage after a health condition required hospitalization.

> My medical insurance was attached [to my job]. They did pay for the hospital stay and when I got out they cancelled me. I had no medical insurance and I could not get the AZT or anything. . . . The medical insurance said that [my HIV-positive status] was preexisting and I had the insurance for 5 years and they canceled me completely. (U.S. gay white male)

Tony also lost his coverage after hospitalization. He said his insurance company went through his records deliberately to find a basis for cutting him off benefits.

> When I got sick and went into the hospital last year, my insurance dropped me, cancelled me. Well . . . I had that particular policy for two years, and when they figured out what was wrong with me, they went back and were looking for some reason to cancel me, and found that I didn't tell them that I had seen a dermatologist when I filled out the application, and they say that I lied. . . . And they didn't just drop me, they rescinded the policy to day one. They didn't cover a thing. They sent me a check of what I paid them for two years. (U.S. gay white male)

These three examples show instances where benefits are abruptly terminated upon hospitalization when they are most needed. People living
with HIV in the United States with good coverage may suddenly find
themselves uninsured if an insurer can determine that they were HIV-
positive before employment at a particular workplace.

People cannot be cut off basic health insurance under the Canadian
plan because of a pre-existing condition. Rick, however, said that he lost
supplementary workplace benefits on the basis of HIV infection predat-
ing employment. He continued to receive basic health coverage from
the government plan, but he was ineligible for the supplementary benefits that included drug, dental, and eye-care plans, as well as life insurance and a long-term disability plan insuring wages in the event of a
medical situation requiring extended leave from work.

> You get your questionnaires to fill out and then like if you have
> HIV they'll disqualify you saying it's a pre-existing condition even
> though you probably worked there for a year. (Canadian gay
> white male)

Workplace benefits plans can raise complex confidentiality issues for
people living with HIV who may be impelled toward the development of
strategies to conceal their diagnosis from insurers (Weitz 1990:32). This
leads people to think twice, for example, about submitting bills for prescription benefit plans. Nick described the lengths to which he went to
keep his HIV-status confidential.

> Initially . . . the doctor, through my request, did not clarify me as HIV-
> positive, because I don't trust any paying institution out there. I asked
> them not to because I don't need any red flags to come up, so I was
> classified with lymphadenopathy, which is, well it could happen to any-
> body. It is not uncommon.

The down side to this kind of strategy is the fear that exposure could
have serious consequences.

> Nothing has been effected, everything has worked out but I have not
> tested the system. I have a fear that it is just going to be wiped away
> from me.

The use of his drug benefits plan could expose his HIV-status.

> I have a prescription rider so any prescriptions that he would write
> would be paid for through my company. Now if I chose to do a drug
> on my own, the company has no knowledge of that. But I would be stu-
> pid not to use a $1.50 prescription rider. I have never had to, and I

think as these last few years have gone on, I am now willing to try. (U.S. gay white male)

The preservation of this "not officially diagnosed" status was a major priority in Andy's health care strategy.

I went to a testing place that's anonymous and confidential so there is no record anywhere of my having a pre-existing condition, which is a big issue. And I had the doctor and I saw him fudge the medical records, which they will do. He wrote in there that he was treating me for fatigue.

Andy was careful to ensure that nothing in his medical record could be construed as grounds for exclusion due to a "pre-existing condition" while attempting to join a medical insurance plan through a new job.

I had the dentist put into my chart that he was treating trench mouth. Trench mouth doesn't flag on insurance companies, where thrush does, so I had to put into the records, trench mouth. . . . If my system will tolerate it, I would prefer to go with Bactrim [for PCP prophylaxis] because it doesn't red flag the insurance company. (U.S. gay white male)

Losing Employment-Related Health Insurance

There are a number of ways, then, that people living with HIV in the United States end up not having medical insurance. People who are uninsured generally cannot afford the regular contact with a doctor essential for the monitoring and anticipation of problems associated with AIDS. Indeed, they are often unable to afford any medical treatment. This can mean that they receive medical attention only in the most dire emergencies, if at all. Wayne had stopped visiting his doctor's despite the doctor's recommendation of monthly visits.

I don't have any insurance right now . . . That scared me at first because I was supposed to go back to the doctor every month. I stopped going to him in June of '89, because I went down twice and it was $700. (U.S. gay white male)

Warren was supposed to be covered for doctor's visits, but he was being billed. As a result, he was staying away from his doctor until he could speak to his social worker about the situation.

That is supposed to be taken care of through Chronic Care but it has been a lot of hassle about . . . my last doctor's appointment, 'cause my case had closed. So I didn't want to go because they send me bills, $50 for a visit. I got to get to my worker. (U.S. gay black male)

Losing employment-related health coverage typically requires a difficult leap into a transitional system of temporary benefits or into privately funded insurance premiums. Ted was committed to maintaining his former workplace plan, even though it was very expensive.

> I have Blue Cross, they haven't cut me from their Blue Cross, and even if they do, the State of Michigan requires that they give me a pick-up policy, much worse benefits but I have already talked to Blue Cross about that. That is already in place. So as soon as they do cut me, I'll be billed individually and it will be very expensive, but what can you do? You can't go without. (U.S. gay white male)

Not everyone was willing to bear the expense. Wayne went uninsured instead.

> They gave you the option of keeping it for 18 months, or whatever, after. They wanted me to pay them so they could turn around and pay the insurance company. I said "no." . . . It was only $150 or so. I didn't like their terms anyway. It didn't cover that much. (U.S. gay white male)

The cost of premiums can be astronomic if an insurance company discovers a client is HIV-positive. Peter left work soon after being diagnosed. He had been tested through his doctor rather than an anonymous clinic and the bill had gone back to the insurance company. As a result, his premiums for maintaining coverage were boosted sharply.

> I hadn't had my test done anonymously. I had had it done through my regular physician, and of course the bill went back for the test. And then some bills came back for some more follow-up tests and then for some more follow-up tests and by that time, the insurance company could figure out what was going on. And by that time I was ready to quit work, which was some ten weeks later. And I went to extend the policy on a personal basis and the premiums had gone up five to ten times. . . . My group rate, they were paying $160 a month and then it went to $1600 a month. (U.S. gay white male)

In addition to the cost of premiums, private insurance plans often contain a copayment so that the user must pay a portion of the bill. Two people told us they faced copayments of 20%.[7] Gordon had a 20% copayment in his policy, but it did not apply to the treatment of chronic conditions. He was saved expenses of about $3,000 a year when the insurer defined AZT as a treatment for a chronic condition.

AZT, I just bought it, my co-pay is 20%. Now our insurance company has said that because it is a chronic type of thing they cover it 100%, but if it wasn't, if I switched to another policy, that is another $2–3,000 a year out of my pocket. Actually I would be a lot more aware of HIV when I was paying $2–3,000 a year, because that would actually impact my day to day living substantially. I mean I just don't have $3,000 to throw away, but that would be the cost. (U.S. heterosexual white male)

Many insurance policies do not provide comprehensive coverage. Clarence had to pay for regular visits to his doctor's office.

I have Blue Cross, Blue Shield. . . . so it covers all the in-hospital expenses and, but as far as the clinic and my doctor, I pay a $100 a month. . . . My doctor visits and a lot of the clinic they don't pay for. . . . (U.S. gay aboriginal/white male)

Jim was fortunate to be covered by his mother's workplace plan. However, he was worried that the cost of regular doctor's visits was adding up.

I have the medical coverage, but it has been bad because Blue Cross doesn't cover office visits and the doctors tell you to come so often. It is really kind of a problem right now, still, all the medical bills. Kind of working on that and hoping something, as far as having a chance to pay some money, to get me out of debt as far as medical expenses, and student loans, hoping something financial come along some day. Every time I go to the doctor it is like $25, $30. (heterosexual black male)

Copayments can add up to the extent that people amass significant medical debts, such as those faced by Dan.

Yea I've got some medical debts that are still hanging around. I just can't afford to pay them, so I don't let them bother me. When they did the lancing, when they cut open my arm about a year ago, and my foot, both of those, I had some health insurance that only covered a portion of it. The rest of it is just too much for me to able to pay, so I haven't paid it. (U.S. gay white male)

In addition to these copayments, people may find themselves paying for specific treatments not covered by their insurance. David mentioned a decision by his insurance company to stop paying for a treatment after covering it for months.

Suddenly something that they have been paying for for six months starts coming through on your hospital bills. We had a case where we were both on aerosol pentamidine. . . . [Partner's] was paid, a covered benefit, and suddenly when I started under Blue Cross, they rejected mine and at the same time they started rejecting his.

The hospital assured him that it was an approved treatment that should be covered by his insurance company.

> You could talk to them and they would say, "Yes, it should be covered, it is on the approved list we don't know why, but it is not." When it comes to the bill not being paid . . . they forgot they ever said that, and they say it is your insurance carrier, and it is your medical bill, you must straighten it out. (U.S. gay white male)

The most consistent problem with the coverage of treatments was payment for prescription medications. This was true both in the United States and Canada. Uninsured people have no coverage for drugs. Bill was not eligible for Medicaid and had to go without medications even though he was getting sicker.

> I got sick in January. They still wouldn't give me Medicaid. They told me no. . . . I got sicker, because I didn't have AZT. . . . It was expensive and I couldn't afford it. So I just didn't take it. So, by the grace of God, I was almost dead. (U.S. gay black male)

Private insurance plans often exclude experimental medications. This may mean that people have to pay for extremely expensive treatments out of their own pockets. Clarence found himself in the position of having to pay for a costly experimental medication.

> [This medication] hasn't been FDA approved yet, so a lot of the insurance companies won't cover it. It's a replacement for Nizoral to clear the thrush. It's very expensive. It's $400 for 20 pills. (U.S. gay aboriginal/white male)

Duane reported large monthly expenditures for medications on top of insurance premiums.

> The premiums aren't that bad, but again it doesn't cover prescription drugs so I spend like $400, $500 a month on prescription drugs. (U.S. gay white male)

There are also drugs that Medicaid does not cover. Kevin said that he had to decide about whether or not he could afford to take medications that were not covered by Medicaid.

> The only problems that I have had was when the doctor writes a prescription that Medicaid doesn't cover. It is a matter of if I want to spend

my own money for that, or if I want to go back to him and tell him to give me something that Medicaid covers. If it is not on the list then you have to pay for it out of your pocket, and sometimes I am not willing to take my limited resources. (U.S. heterosexual black male)[8]

Medication costs affect Canadian and U.S. study participants in similar ways because both have to rely on supplementary workplace plans or specific income assistance programs (Smith 1994). The absence of drug plan coverage forces people to find creative ways of obtaining medications. One of these is to share drugs, so that people who do not have coverage obtain medications from people who do (Weitz 1991:87). Andy was uninsured and relied on his insured friends for a variety of medications.

> I have not had insurance coverage since . . . I lost my job in August, so I've been getting most of the medications I've been using through friends of mine. I've been getting my AZT, I've been getting Motrin, I've been getting sinus medication, I've been getting it from friends of mine.

He was trying to get involved in clinical trials to obtain medications.

> Now I think my T-cells are probably low enough that I can qualify for studies. I'm looking into a study at Harper Hospital that's a combination AZT-DDI. I really want to get into that because my main thrust now is looking at extending the period of time. It's so damn stupid and it makes me so angry that I go for a study and they say, "Well yeah, your Ts have to be below 200," and I say, "Well, then you've got opportunistic infections setting in so what you want is people at death's door essentially." It gets me so angry that the protocols are so rigid you can't possibly fit into them. (U.S. gay white male)

These are creative responses to the limitations of the health care system in providing access to necessary medications. It does, however, point to a real problem with drug costs that threatens the health of people living with HIV in both the United States and Canada.

Going on Medicaid

People who are not employed need to meet quite specific conditions to be eligible for full medical coverage through Medicaid in the United States. There are often long waits and quite stringent restrictions in terms of financial considerations and health status. This means that many people are caught in a state of limbo waiting for coverage. Bill

found that he could not get proper health care coverage until he was
extremely ill.

> But once they thought I was going to die, it was like Medicaid here you
> go. But before that it was like, "No, you don't get anything." . . . And I
> watch people go through that today. Before they can get Medicaid,
> they have to go through so much illness. (U.S. gay black male)

Devon was sufficiently ill to be unable to carry on with his job and yet did
not meet the criteria for an AIDS diagnosis. He applied a number of
times before being accepted for benefits.

> The way it has been, the only people that were approved for social
> security and disability were those that had AIDS. But I was so close to it,
> having all the symptoms that I could no longer do my regular work
> that I was educated and trained in, nor could I do any physical labor.
> I was denied twice social security and I had to reapply. Like I said, it has
> been two years . . . (U.S. gay black male)

The wait to qualify for Medicaid meant that Bob was forced to keep paying premiums to maintain coverage while living on Social Security.

> I finally just got Social Security but I think there is going to be a need
> for me to work part time if I want to keep up my private Blue Cross,
> Green Shield which is like $300 a month. . . . I have been paying my
> own premiums. [His previous employer] paid for a certain period of
> time. . . . You have to wait two years from the disability to get on the
> better programs [Medicare]. It's real screwy. (U.S. gay white male)

Devon was in the process of "spending down" in order to qualify for
Medicaid. He was having trouble obtaining medical services because of
the unpaid bills he was accumulating and had to rely on the good will of
his doctor to continue receiving medical attention.

> Now I have this Medicaid spend down, where you have to accrue a cer-
> tain amount of medical expenses before you are issued medical cover-
> age. It is a headache. . . . I can't make my appointments, I can't get my
> prescriptions, because I already owe a $1000 in medical expenses that
> have not been paid. . . . I am just thankful that I have a good doctor.
> She knows that she will get paid for her services. That is the frustrating
> part. It goes back to where we were talking about earlier, having to
> depend on other people. I am not used to this. (U.S. gay black male)

Wayne described the process of impoverishment to which he was
subjected.

They can't touch your house, but your car is an asset, my IRAs, a little
money in the bank, not much, it's going fast. I was living off my savings.
Now it is going down to nothing, but that is OK with me.

An AIDS service organization had advised him to let medical bills build
up in order to qualify for Medicaid. U.S. residents may be put in
the position of having to leave their jobs in order to qualify for effective medical coverage. Carl had to leave work in order to be eligible
for Medicaid.

I ended up having to legally not work, to get the medical attention I
needed because I'm not insured. (U.S. gay white male)

In comparison, the universal coverage provided in the Canadian health
care system means that people with HIV can work longer and retain their
belongings without sacrificing basic medical treatment.

In Michigan there are a few other options for people who are not
employed and do not qualify for Medicaid. The state will temporarily
pick up the cost of paying premiums for some people to continue with
the medical insurance plan associated with previous employment. David
benefitted from this program.

[In] Michigan, the state had a pilot program and they decided it
would save them an awful lot of money. . . . If you are unemployed and
cannot pay . . . it is much cheaper for the state of Michigan to pay your
insurance payment than it is to pick you up on Medicaid. So there is a
program. You have to apply for it and they will pay your insurance premiums for eighteen months. It was master medical, Blue Cross, Blue
Shield, so I didn't have a problem with that, other than . . . it was in
jeopardy because I lost my job. (U.S. gay white male)

Andy did not take advantage of this program because it required disclosure of his HIV-positive status.

Now the state of Michigan has a program where they will pick up the
cost of your insurance premiums because it's cheaper than paying for
your health care. So they'll pick them up but you have to be officially
diagnosed and I'm not officially diagnosed. (U.S. gay white male)

An "official" diagnosis carried two serious costs that outweighed the benefit of the short-term plan. It would have invalidated his life insurance
policy so that his funeral expenses would no longer be covered and it
would have labeled him with a "pre-existing" condition preventing any
further eligibility for health coverage.

Others were either unaware of this program or ineligible for it. Tony applied for insurance but found the premiums would amount to about $6,000 a year. As result, he was uninsured.

> To get another insurance I did get, I applied to Blue Cross and Blue Shield, which is the big major one, and they will insure me, but it is almost $500 a month. Well if I am going to pay that much, and then there is a year waiting . . . period before they cover anything, so you pay the premiums for a year and then they will take you in and start picking things up. If I am going to be putting out $500 a month, I may as well be paying my own bills. (U.S. gay white male)

In addition to premium assistance, there are local programs in Michigan that provide a lesser level of health care to people ineligible for Medicaid. Two participants had been covered by County Care, one of these local programs. County Care has a reputation as a "second class" system made available only to the indigent. It offers access to treatment only at specified clinics and lacks the staff or resources for adequate service. Lemuel described that service:

> At first I had County Care, which is a crapola system. They select twenty little pill pushing clinics you go to and the doctor and even the pharmacist, dentist, all of it. And [his doctor] wasn't in that package, and I had to get referrals from this clinic to go to [this doctor], which was a lot of trouble and a lot of BS. (U.S. gay black male)

Andrea was disturbed at the length of time it took to get prescriptions filled through the County Care system.

> Over at this County Care you are set at a certain program, you have to go to certain doctors, which is the same with the HMO. . . . Before, I could go to any pharmacy, they had to call up and get it approved before they could fill it out for me and that took like 3 or 4 hours. So now I know that when I do start running low I have to make my appointment at least a month ahead of time, to give me those days that it is going to take them. (U.S. heterosexual black female)

Andrea was able to compensate for the limitation of County Care through sharing her fiancé's medications. Her fiancé was on Medicaid.

The labyrinthine tangle of rules governing health care eligibility in the United States, the ease by which insurers can exclude patients, and the interaction of employment and access to health care fosters an environment that demands advanced skills in trouble shooting. Many U.S. HIV-positive people have considerable knowledge in negotiating with bureaucracies. They may, as well, develop arrangements with their physicians for "rule bending" in order to secure basic health care, or enter into informal drug economies where people with insurance help out friends and acquaintances with medications that they have on hand but no longer need.

Conclusion

Place of residence clearly differentiates the experience of gaining access to health care among the study participants. Few other areas of life affected by HIV could be distinguished by nationality. Seropositive people offer a grassroots perspective on the impact of social organization upon people who are ill. The fundamental difference is evident in the simple fact that Canadians had little to say about their access to health care, as they could take it as a matter of course, while U.S. residents had a great deal to say about their many struggles around securing basic treatment. Some U.S. respondents have no health insurance as a result of being unemployed and are thus ineligible for government plans, because of working in a job without benefits, or because of exclusion from plans due to a "pre-existing condition." Many of those who have succeeded in being included in medical plans face copayments, heavy premiums that can escalate suddenly because of an HIV diagnosis, limitations on treatments, and the threat that coverage may suddenly be eliminated when it is most needed. Further, many U.S. insurance plans are now placing limits on total insurability, meaning that an individual can be terminated after exceeding a certain threshold of health care expenditure.

While current government budgetary crises threaten the continuation of public, universal health care in Canada, the experiences of people with HIV disease show clearly that the public system functions far better in providing access to uninterrupted medical care without prematurely forcing recipients out of work or into poverty. The privately organized, corporate system, in contrast, functions least well in providing medical services to people who most need health care, and who are in low-wage or insecure job sectors that are less likely to be unionized or to have health insurance benefit plans. The AIDS epidemic in the United States has struck especially hard among black people, Latinos, and (other) people who have long suffered economic marginalization. This has meant that the U.S. health care system has been particularly badly prepared to deal with the consequences of AIDS, and that a major portion of the distress suffered by people with HIV has been inflicted by (rather than alleviated by) the health care system itself. The U.S. system very often inflicts an agonizing process of impoverishment on people with life-threatening illnesses and on their families as well at a time when they are severely stressed by the effects of illness itself (Corbin and Strauss 1988:112). It also means that these problems have proven to be particularly intractable because neither racial minority groups, gay people, poor people, nor drug users have had sufficient economic or political influence to bring about a change that would not only benefit them but would also improve the health of Americans as a whole. Despite the impressive work of AIDS movement organizations, which have revolutionized the ways in which AIDS has been perceived (Adam 1996), the persistent reinforcement of notions of "innocent" and "deserving victims" by the media, courts, and governments has continually absolved U.S. society of its responsibility in exacerbating the plight of people with HIV.

CONCLUSION

Steve Levitt's 1994 short film *Deaf Heaven* portrays a man searching for a sense of place amidst the maelstrom of AIDS while attending to his dying lover in hospital. The film raises many of the issues that press upon any caring observer of AIDS including survivor's guilt, existential anxiety, and the search for meaning amid tragic absurdity. At a moment when his lover has drifted into sleep, the central character of the film encounters an old man in the hospital who recounts the loss of his family in Auschwitz and names the role he has been cast in by history. The old man says he is an *eydes* or witness fated to preserve and re-tell the story of the Holocaust in the present. His loss and suffering have meaning, then, even if he found himself to be a virtually helpless, and unheroic, observer unable to change the course of events.

We found, in several instances, that people with AIDS formulated a similar role for us as researchers, looking to us to witness their lives (an experience reported as well by Rose Weitz [1987] and, in the context of other life-threatening diseases, by Arthur Kleinman [1988:xii, 10]). Study participants sought to use us as a sounding board for confronting the terror of HIV and for organizing the meaning of HIV in their lives. Many were eager to accept our offer to help act as a medium for communicating their accumulated experience to other people touched by AIDS. While we could scarcely offer adequate answers or take on the full enormity of bearing witness, our interest has been to do research that accepts some of these larger implications.

The established scientific model constructs a series of barricades against its subjects by distancing them through standardized tests, turning them into numbers as if they lack social analyses of their own, and positing them as objects for administrative manipulation—all in the name of objectivity. Our resistance to this model and willingness to explore the subjectivity of HIV disease alarmed several grant reviewers who were convinced that people with HIV would be in such a fragile psychological state that they would be easily shattered by the interview process. Reviewers' anxieties mirrored the social taboos often shared by respondents' families and friends who tiptoed around issues that people in the syndrome put considerable thought and energy into solving. As should be clear from the preceding chapters, the participants in this study were very much interested in articulating their concerns to someone who wanted to hear their opinions and perceptions. Like us, Barbara Giacquinta (1989:35) and Juliet Corbin and Anselm Strauss (1988:290) found the people they interviewed to be fully capable and eager to talk.

To use the language of phenomenological and discourse theories, this study sought to bracket a series of positivist presumptions about "personality" in order to see how the subject positions of seropositivity traverse a problematic social landscape, negotiate and construct the real, and rework socially available AIDS discourses. We made no presumptions about "stages" of dying (see Kessler, Price and Wortman 1985:537). And we hoped through research to help empower seropositive people and their caregivers in the sense that

> to be empowered is not only to speak in one's own voice and to tell one's own story, but to apply the understanding arrived at to action in accord with one's own interests (Mishler 1986:119; see also Cannon 1989:64; Viney and Bousfield 1991:757).

Our concern has been to capture an interactive and moving process and thus to contribute toward a culture of living with HIV. It has been, as well, an interest in seeing how discourses are deployed to organize, make sense of, and construct experiences around HIV, recognizing that this encoding process occurs in a politicized social environment where interpretive systems are thrust upon seropositive people from many directions and by powerful institutional sources.

Active Coping

While a number of general schema have been proposed to characterize the concerns and coping strategies developing around HIV disease (Sandstrom 1990; Siegel and Krauss 1991; Getzel 1991; O'Brien 1992:162–171; Schwartzberg 1993), the greatest interest among researchers of coping with disease has centered around so-called "active-cognitive" coping (Nerenz and Leventhal 1983:26–28; Namir et al. 1987:317). A good deal of research on cancer (Weisman 1979:23), as well as HIV (Leserman, Perkins and Evans 1992; Kurdek and Siesky 1990; Rabkin et al. 1990), concludes that active coping with illness is associated with higher quality of life, less depression, and an enhanced sense of well-being. By contrast, avoidance, passivity, or resignation appear to be part of a larger syndrome of hopelessness and anxiety. Wolf et al. (1991:172) found:

> Active-cognitive coping was significantly related to lower total mood disturbance and depression as well as increased vigor. . . . Avoidance coping was significantly related to greater depression and lower vigor.

William Nicholson and Bonita Long (1990:874) report in addition that

> greater internalized homophobia (. . .) and poorer self-esteem (. . .) are associated with the relatively greater use of avoidant coping. . . . whereas worry about one's health (. . .) and a positive attitude toward homosexuality (. . .) are associated with greater proactive coping.

Research on cancer suggests that active, resistive approaches to illness may even be associated with longer survival time (Coates, Temoshok and Mandel 1984; Solomon and Temoshok 1987). Whether greater longevity is attainable or not, learning from those who have already been dealing with problems may, at least, help develop personal repertoires of strategies or recipes for dealing with HIV-related difficulties.

AIDS in Transition

In the decade and a half since its identification in the medical literature, AIDS has been re-shaped as it has been taken up by shifting public discourses. In the early 1980s, the ominous spread of the epidemic met silence and official indifference (Adam 1992a,c). The "pioneers," as one participant referred to people diagnosed at that time, often had to make their own way through the health care system and social services, assisted only through their personal social networks (friends, families, and lovers). Silence gave way to panic and blame in the mid-1980s as "family values" supporters tried to seize AIDS as a moral weapon to wield against critics of sexual and gender inequality.

The advances won since then have not simply been handed down by benevolent governments and caring communities. They have been fought for and won by a movement made up of a variety of organizations, including gay and lesbian groups, community service agencies, organizations run by and for people living with AIDS and HIV, and groups arising from and serving specific communities. Collectively these organizations have chalked up remarkable achievements, whether in the form of the development of new services, significant changes in government policy, or important alterations in the public face of AIDS.

Many of the resources the participants in this study deployed result from the activities of the AIDS movement. People entering the syndrome now can find a great deal of useful information regarding the medical and social aspects of life with HIV, connect to case management services, or join support groups to pool experiences. At the same time, the maze of government services and benefits has been made more accessible through the advocacy work of AIDS organizations and important precedents set by "pioneers" demanding needed assistance. There are still important gaps in these services, and people have variable access to them depending on such factors as location, ethnicity, gender, sexual orientation, or social class. Nevertheless, they comprise an important set of resources that make a real difference in the lives of the diverse aggregation of people living with AIDS and HIV who participated in this study.

Yet these gains remain vulnerable in the face of the neoconservative agenda which has swept the jurisdictions where the participants in this study live. Some of the participants have already been affected by the attacks on general welfare assistance undertaken by the Engler administration in Michigan and the Harris government in Ontario since the interviews took place. Of the 60 HIV-positive participants in this study, 37 were not employed at the time we spoke with them. Some of these were on disability benefits of various kinds; others depended on general welfare programs to survive. As cutbacks reach deeper into child care services, educational institutions, public transit (including transportation for the disabled), and health care programs the choices available to people living with HIV and AIDS narrow substantially.

Further, this political shift to the right has been accomplished in part through the use of a moral agenda which has blamed people receiving welfare benefits, people of color, immigrants, women, and gay people for a variety of contemporary social problems. At present, people with

AIDS and HIV are affected insofar as they are poor (and many of the participants in this study are, as discussed in chapter 5) or unhealthy. Neoconservative rhetoric has already laid a trap for AIDS programs precisely because the people most affected by AIDS are the people already targeted as "undeserving."

This book has emphasized the ways in which people make lives for themselves in the face of the challenges and barriers imposed by HIV and AIDS. It is a record of courage and creativity as well as mistakes and missed opportunities. People make lives for themselves, however, in specific historical circumstances with particular resources at hand. Many of the participants in this study were just scraping by on a meager basis. They are highly vulnerable to reversals if these resources are diminished. This is the next challenge facing the AIDS movement and its allies.

NOTES

Preface

1. In 1991, the Business Meeting of the American Sociological Association passed the following resolution:

GIVEN THAT
1. In 1990, Congress repealed legislation that barred HIV-antibody positive visitors to the United States and passed new legislation which placed responsibility for designating disease which could result in banning in the hands of the Public Health Service,
2. The enforcement of bans against HIV-antibody positive persons is arbitrary and demeaning, falling heavily on AIDS educators and activists carrying AIDS-related material over the border because, practically speaking, seropositive people cannot be recognized by immigration officials,
3. Discriminatory legislation led to an international boycott of the Sixth World Congress on AIDS held in San Francisco and the cancellation of the Eighth World Congress which was to be held in Boston,
4. The United States has the greatest number of HIV-antibody positive people in the world and has few grounds to regard itself as threatened by the importation of HIV,
5. The ban against HIV-antibody positive visitors to the United States is universally condemned by the International AIDS Society, by public

health officials, and by workers and activists on the front lines of the battle against AIDS,

6. The ban represents an unnecessary and harmful violation of the right to free movement by people living with HIV disease, and in particular, results in their being restricted in doing work and research around AIDS, and

7. The Sociologists' AIDS Network finds the ban of no value in the prevention of AIDS and that it is positively harmful to research on AIDS and to the lives of people with AIDS and HIV,

THEREFORE MOVED THAT

The President of the American Sociological Association communicate to President Bush, to the Secretary of Health and Human Services, to the Public Health Service, to the Centres for Disease Control, and to the International AIDS Society our recommendation that the ban on HIV-antibody positive visitors to the United States be lifted immediately.

Introduction

1. The expression "present at their own making" is taken from Thompson (1968:8).

2. Alzheimer's Disease was at first applied only to younger people with symptoms of senility (presenile dementia) as memory loss among the elderly was taken for granted. It took a change of definition to count memory loss among the elderly as an illness (see Deboni and McLachlan 1980).

3. This reorganization of meanings can occur at the cultural as well as the individual level, so that illness can operate, in Susan Sontag's (1978) famous formulation, as a metaphor.

4. Peter Leonard (1984:180—201) discusses the complexities of marginalization in contemporary capitalist society and its connection with intensified subordination and damaged self-concepts.

5. On Cameron (1993), see Adam (Forthcoming).

6. The story of AIDS activism is told in Watney (1987), Gamson (1989), Kramer (1989), Patton (1990a,b), Kinsman (1992), and Adam (1996).

7. Several seropositive respondents were also caregivers to other HIV-positive friends, lovers, or spouses.

8. Rose Weitz's (1991) study *Life With AIDS* is a notable exception to this pattern, having been done in Arizona.

9. These two participants have been allocated according to their second-stated ethnicity in the chart below. As well, several U.S. participants indicated Canadian parentage; similarly some Canadians mentioned American heritage.

10. Barbara Giacquinta (1989:35) reports a similar experience.

1. In the Beginning

1. All names used here are pseudonyms. Pseudonyms are used consistently so that all statements attributed to the same name do refer to the same person.

2. AIDS Related Complex, a term which has fallen into disuse, describes minor symptoms of HIV infection.

3. Discourse and Identity

1. The next five paragraphs draw on Adam (1996).
2. George Getzel (1991) has also formulated a meaning typology based on phenomenological principles. This inventory typifies personalities rather than meanings *per se* as follows: the "beneficent type," "the heroic type," the "artistic-spiritual type," and the "rational-instrumental type." Similarly, Diane Ragsdale, Joseph Kotarba, and James Morrow (1994) typologize coping in terms of the following personalities: loner, medic, time keeper, activist, mystic, and victim.
3. This politic is common in public discourse on women and AIDS. See especially Corea (1992).

4. Sex and Love

1. The "you" in this instance refers to two other women who were also being interviewed at the same time.
2. This theme appears in the form of Greek statuary on the cover of Paul Monette's (1988) *Borrowed Time*, a memoir of the death of a man from AIDS written by his lover.
3. Levine and Siegel (1992:63) report a similar finding in their investigation of unprotected sexual practices.

5. Family and Friends

1. This view usually comes up as part of a therapeutic discourse, discussed in chapter 3.
2. Fortunately many of the women we interviewed spoke highly of a women's shelter and an outreach agency in Detroit, both of which provided support specifically for HIV-positive mothers.

6. Working

1. There were three who did not respond to the question.
2. This organizational approach underlies Barr, Waring and Warshaw (1991); Emery and Puckett (1988); Masi (1990); Patterson (1989); and Tedlow and Marram (1991).
3. Paul Bellaby (1990) discusses the tension between work-discipline and illness.
4. In this study, participants in Ontario were protected by the inclusion of sexual orientation in the provincial human rights code. In Michigan, they were not. At the time of this study, seven of the ten Canadian provinces and seven of the fifty states forbid discrimination on the basis of sexual orientation.
5. The American trade union movement has lost considerable ground over the past twenty years, as measured in memberships, strength at the bargaining table, or political influence. The Canadian labor movement is in a relatively stronger position in the early 1990s. Union membership is higher in Canada and Canadian unions are more likely to take up social issues than their American counterparts. (See Schenk and Bernard 1992, Morand 1992, and Navarro 1992).

6. See Vogel (1990) for a useful look at workplace strategies concerning pregnant women.

7. Experiencing Health Care in Two Nations

1. Patricia Butler (1988:75) describes the United States as the only industrialized nation without a national health program with the exception of South Africa.

2. Daniel Fife and James McAnaney (1993:516) explain that "pre-existing condition" clauses can also be invoked when an employer changes insurers to exclude even people continuing at the same workplace whose illness predates the new policy.

3. Studies by John Fleshman and Vincent Mor (1993), Jesse Green and Peter Arno (1990) and Nancy Kass et al. (1991) also discuss the problems posed by loss of private insurance among people living with HIV infection.

4. Marilyn Ellwood et al. (1991:1043) found that more than two thirds of the people living with AIDS who were covered by Medicaid in California and more than one third of those in New York were classified as medically needy on the basis of spend down. The proportion who qualified as medically needy is smaller in New York as the higher infection rate among the urban poor in that state means that more people living with HIV already meet the poverty criteria.

5. Of those who mentioned being on Medicaid, 12 are black and 5 white; 5 are female and 12 male.

6. While coverage of same-sex partners is increasingly common in union contracts in Canada, none of the Canadian participants in this study had a partner with such benefits.

7. Ted and Terry also had to make copayments covering 20% of expenses.

8. Three other participants—Dan, Duane, and Frank—also reported problems with medications not being covered by Medicaid.

REFERENCES

Adam, Barry D. 1978. *The Survival of Domination.* New York: Elsevier/
Greenwood.

Adam, Barry D. 1992a. "The State, Public Policy and AIDS Discourse." In
James Miller, ed. *Fluid Exchanges.* Toronto: University of Toronto Press.

Adam, Barry D. 1992b. "Sociology and People Living with AIDS." In Joan
Huber and Beth Schneider, eds. *The Social Context of AIDS.* Newbury
Park, CA: Sage.

Adam, Barry D. 1992c. "Sex and Caring Among Men." In Kenneth
Plummer, ed., *Modern Homosexualities,* pp. 175–183. London:
Routledge.

Adam, Barry D. 1996. "Mobilizing Around AIDS." In John Gagnon, Peter
Nardi, and Martin Levine, eds. *In Changing Times.* Chicago: University
of Chicago.

Adam, Barry D. Forthcoming. Miriam Cameron. "Living With AIDS."
Disability Studies Quarterly.

Adam, Barry D and Alan Sears. 1994. "Negotiating sexual relationships
after testing HIV-positive." *Medical Anthropology* 16:63–77.

Adam, Barry D and Alan Sears. 1994. *People with HIV/AIDS Talk . . .
About Life, Love, Work, and Family.* Windsor, Ontario: AIDS Committee
of Windsor.

Altman, Dennis. 1986. *AIDS in the Mind of America*. Garden City, NY: Doubleday.

Anderson, Veanne. 1992. "For Whom Is this World Just?" *Journal of Applied Social Psychology* 22 (3):248–259.

Atkinson, J., et al. 1988. "The Prevalence of Psychiatric Disorders Among Men with Human Immunodeficiency Virus." *Archives of General Psychiatry* 45 (9):859–864.

Barr, Judith, Joan Waring, and Leon Warshaw. 1991. "Employees Sources of AIDS Information." *Journal of Occupational Medicine* 33 (2):143–147.

Becker, Ernest. 1971. *The Birth and Death of Meaning*. New York: Free Press.

Bellaby, Paul. 1990. "What is 'Genuine' Sickness?" *Sociology of Health and Illness* 12 (1):47–68.

Berliner, Howard S. 1977. "Emerging Ideologies in Medicine." *Review of Radical Political Economics* 9 (1): 103–122.

Bérubé, Allan. 1988. "Caught in the Storm." *Out/Look* 1 (3):8.

Billingsley, Andrew. 1973. "Black Families and White Social Science." In Joyce Ladner, ed., *The Death of White Sociology*. New York: Vintage.

Bodenheimer, Thomas. 1992. "Underinsurance in America." *New England Journal of Medicine* 327 (4):274–277.

Bor, Robert, Riva Miller, and Eleanor Goldman. 1993. "HIV/AIDS and the Family." *Journal of Family Therapy* 15:187–204.

Britton, P. J., J. J. Zarski, and S. E. Hobfoll. 1993. "Psychological Distress and the Role of Significant Others in a Population of Gay/Bisexual Men in the Era of HIV." *AIDS Care* 5 (1):43–54.

Brown, Marie, and Gail Powell-Cope. 1991. "AIDS Family Caregiving" *Nursing Research* 40 (6):338–345.

Brown, Marie, and Gail Powell-Cope. 1992. *Caring for a Loved One with AIDS*. Seattle: University of Washington.

Bury, Judy. 1994. "Women and the AIDS Epidemic" In J. Bury and S. McLachlan, eds. *Women and the AIDS Epidemic*. London: Routledge.

Bury, Michael. 1982. "Chronic Illness as Biographical Disruption." *Sociology of Health and Illness* 4 (2): 167–182.

Bury, Michael. 1988. "Social Constructionism and the Development of Medical Sociology." *Sociology of Health and Illness* 8 (2):137–169.

Butler, Patricia. 1988. *Too Poor To Be Sick*. Washington, D.C.: American Public Health Association.

Cameron, Miriam. 1993. *Living With AIDS*. Newbury Park, CA: Sage.

Cannon, Sue. 1989. "Social Research in Stressful Settings." *Sociology of Health and Illness* 11 (1):62–77.

Carter, Erica and Simon Watney. 1989. *Taking Liberties*. London: Serpent's Tail.

Cates, Jim et al. 1990. "The Effects of AIDS on the Family System." *Families in Society* 71 (4):195–201.

Charmaz, Kathy. 1991. *Good Days, Bad Days*. New Brunswick, NJ: Rutgers University Press.

Clatts, Michael. 1994. "All the King's Horses and All the King's Men." *Human Organization* 53 (1):93–95.

Clatts, Michael, and Kevin Mutchler. 1989. "AIDS and the Dangerous Other." *Medical Anthropology* 10:105–114.

Cleveland, Peggy et al. 1988. "If Your Child Had Aids . . . : Responses of Parents with Homosexual Children." *Family Relations* 37:150.

Coates, Thomas, Lydia Temoshok, and Jeffrey Mandel. 1984. "Psychosocial Research is Essential to Understanding and Treating AIDS." *American Psychologist* 39 (11):1309.

Connell, R. W. et al. 1988. "Social Aspects of the Prevention of AIDS: Study A—Report No. 1, Method and Sample." Sydney, Australia: Macquarie University.

Connors, John, and Patrick Heaven. 1990. "Belief in a Just World and Attitudes Toward AIDS Sufferers." *Journal of Social Psychology* 130 (4):559–560.

Corbin, Juliet, and Anselm Strauss. 1988. *Unending Work and Care*. San Francisco: Jossey-Bass.

Corea, Gena. 1992. *The Invisible Epidemic*. New York: HarperCollins.

Crimp, Douglas. 1988. *AIDS: Cultural Analysis, Cultural Activism*. Cambridge: MIT Press.

Cuthbert, Melinda. 1992. "A Population in Peril." Presented to the Society for the Study of Social Problems Pittsburgh.

DeBoni, Ugo, and Donald McLachlan. 1980. "Senile Dementia and Alzheimer's Disease." *Life Sciences* 27: 1–14.

Denneny, Michael. 1979. *Lovers*. New York: St Martin's.

Denzin, Norman. 1990. "Harold and Agnes." *Sociological Theory* 8 (2):198–216.

Doll, Lynda et al. 1991. "Male Bisexuality and AIDS in the United States." In Rob Tielman, Manuel Carballo and Aart Hendriks, eds. *Bisexuality & HIV/AIDS*. Buffalo: Prometheus.

Doll, Lynda et al. 1992. "Homosexually and Nonhomosexually Identified Men Who Have Sex with Men." *Journal of Sex Research* 29 (1):1–14.

Doyal, Lesley. 1979. *The Political Economy of Health*. London: Pluto.

Ellwood, Marilyn, Thomas Fanning, and Suzanne Dodds. 1991. "Medicaid Eligibility Patterns for Persons with AIDS in California and New York, 1982–87" *Journal of Acquired Immune Deficiency Syndrome* 4:1036–45.

Emery, Alan, and Sam Puckett. 1988. *Managing AIDS in the Workplace*. Reading, Mass.: Addison-Wesley.

Farmer, Paul, and Arthur Kleinman. 1989. "AIDS as Human Suffering." *Daedalus* 118 (2):135–160.

172   References

Fife, Daniel, and James McAnaney. 1993. "Private Medical Insurance
Among Philadelphia Residents Diagnosed with AIDS." *Journal of
Acquired Immune Deficiency Syndrome* 6:512–17.
Fleshman, John, and Vincent Mor. 1993. "Insurance Status Among People
with AIDS." *Inquiry* 30:180–88.
Fox, Alan. 1980. "The Meaning of Work." In G. Esland and G. Salaman,
eds. *The Politics of Work and Occupations.* Toronto: University of
Toronto Press.
Franks, Peter; Carolyn Clancy, and Marthe Gold. 1993. "Health
Insurance and Mortality." *Journal of the American Medical Association*
270 (6):737–41.
Frierson, Robert, Steven Lippmann, and Janet Johnson. 1987. "AIDS:
Psychological Stresses on the Family." *Psychosomatics* 28 (2):65.
Furnham, Adrian, and Edward Procter. 1989. "Belief in a Just World."
British Journal of Social Psychology 28 (4):365–384.
Gamson, Josh. 1989. "Silence, Death, and the Invisible Enemy." *Social
Problems* 36 (4):351–367.
Getzel, George. 1991. "Survival Modes for People with AIDS in Groups."
Social Work 36 (1):7–11.
Giacquinta, Barbara. 1989. "Researching the Effects of AIDS on Families."
American Journal of Hospice Care (May/June):31.
Glennon, Frank, and Stephen Joseph. 1993. "Just World Beliefs, Self-
esteem, and Attitudes Towards Homosexuals with AIDS." *Psychological
Reports* 72 (2):584–586.
Gostin, Lawrence. 1993. "What's Wrong with the ERISA Vacuum?" *Journal
of the American Medical Association* 269 (19):2527–2532.
Green, Jesse, and Peter Arno. 1990. "The 'Medicalization' of AIDS."
Journal of the American Medical Association 264 (10):1261–1266.
Grimshaw, Jonathan. 1989. "The Individual Challenge." In Erica Carter
and Simon Watney, eds. *Taking Liberties.* London: Serpent's Tail.
Hassin, Jeanette. 1994. "Living a Responsible Life." *Social Science and
Medicine* 39 (3):391–400.
Hays, Robert, Sarah Chauncey, and Linda Tobey. 1990. "The Social
Support Networks of Gay Men with AIDS." *Journal of Community
Psychology* 18:374–385.
Heidegger, Martin. 1962. *Being and Time.* New York: Harper & Row.
Herek, Gregory. 1990. "Illness, Stigma, and AIDS." In P. Costa and G.
VandenBos, eds. *Psychological Aspects of Serious Illness.* Washington, D.C.:
American Psychological Association.
Hunter, Nan. 1995. "Complications of Gender." In Beth Schneider
and Nancy Stoller, eds. *Women Resisting AIDS.* Philadelphia: Temple
University Press.
Interrante, Joseph. 1987. "To Have Without Holding." *Radical America* 20:6.

Joseph, J., et al. 1990. "Psychological Functioning in a Cohort of Gay Men At Risk for AIDS." *Journal of Nervous and Mental Disease* 178 (10):607–615.

Kass, Nancy, Ruth Faden, Robin Fox, and Jan Dudley. 1991. "The Loss of Private Health Insurance Among Homosexual Men with AIDS." *Inquiry* 28:249–254.

Kayal, Philip. 1993. *Bearing Witness*. Boulder, CO: Westview.

Kelly, James and Pamelia Sykes. 1989. "Helping the Helpers." *Social Work* 34 (3):239.

Kessler, Ronald, Richard Price and Camille Wortman. 1985. "Social Factors in Psychopathology." *Annual Review of Psychology* 36:531.

Kinsman, Gary. 1992. "Managing AIDS Organizing." In William Carroll, ed., *Organizing Dissent*. Toronto: Garamond.

Kleinman, Arthur. 1988. *The Illness Narratives*. New York: Basic Books.

Kramer, Larry. 1989. *Reports from the Holocaust*. New York: St. Martins.

Kurdek, Lawrence, and Gene Siesky. 1990. "The Nature and Correlates of Psychological Adjustment in Gay Men with AIDS-related Conditions." *Journal of Applied Social Psychology* 20 (10):846–860.

Lamm, Steven, and T. Ford Brewer. 1990. "AIDS in the Workplace." *American Industrial Hygiene Association Journal* 5 (1):736–737.

Land, Helen and George Harangody. 1990. "A Support Group for Partners of Persons with AIDS." *Families in Society* 71 (8):471–482.

Lebowitz, Michael. 1992. *Beyond Capital*. New York: St. Martin's Press.

Leonard, Peter. 1984. *Personality and Ideology*. London: MacMillan.

Leserman, Jane, Diana Perkins, and Dwight Evans. 1992. "Coping with the Threat of AIDS." *American Journal of Psychiatry* 149 (11):1514–1519.

Levine, Carol. 1991. "AIDS and Changing Concepts of Family." In Dorothy Nelkin, David Willis, and Scott Parris, eds. *A Disease of Society*. New York: Cambridge University Press.

Levine, Carol and Ronald Bayer. 1989. "The Ethics of Screening for Early Intervention in HIV Disease." *American Journal of Public Health* 79 (12):1661–1667.

Levine, Martin and Karolynn Siegel. 1992. "Unprotected Sex." In Joan Huber and Beth Schneider, eds. *The Social Context of AIDS*. Newbury Park, CA: Sage.

Lewis, Diane. 1993. "Living with the Threat of AIDS." In Barbara Bair and Susan Cayleff, eds. *Wings of Gauze*. Detroit: Wayne State University Press.

Lovejoy, Nancy. 1990. "AIDS: Impact on the Gay Man's Homosexual and Heterosexual Families." *Marriage and Family Review* 14 (3/4):285–316.

Maj, Mario. 1991. "Psychological Problems of Families and Health Workers Dealing with People Infected with Human Immunodeficiency Virus 1." *Acta Psychiatrica Scandinavica* 83 (1):161–168.

Marzuk, Peter, Helen Tierney, Kenneth Tardiff, Elliot Gross, Leonard Morgan, Ming-Ann Hsu and J. John Mann. 1988. "Increased Risk of

Suicide in Persons with AIDS." *Journal of the American Medical Association* 259 (9):1333–1337.

Masi, Dale. 1990. *AIDS Issues in the Workplace*. Wesport, CT.: Quorum.

McCann, K., and E. Wadsworth. 1992. "The Role of Informed Carers in Supporting Gay Men Who Have HIV Related Illness." *AIDS Care* 4 (1):25–34.

McCormack, Thomas P. 1990. *The AIDS Benefits Handbook*. New Haven: Yale University Press.

Mishler, Elliot. 1986. *Research Interviewing*. Cambridge: Harvard University Press.

Monette, Paul. 1988. *Borrowed Time*. San Diego: Harcourt Brace Jovanovich.

Morand, Martin. 1992. "U.S. and Canadian Labor: A Convergence at Whose Expense?" *Monthly Review* 43: 15–28.

Murphy, Patrice, and Kathleen Perry. 1988. "Hidden Grievers." *Death Studies* 12 (5/6):451.

Namir, S., D. Wolcott, F. Fawzy, and M. Alumbaugh. 1987. "Coping with AIDS." *Journal of Applied Social Psychology* 17 (3):309–328.

Navarro, Vincent. 1992. *Why the United States Does Not Have a National Health Program*. Amityville, N.Y.: Baywood.

Nelkin, Dorothy. 1987. "AIDS and the Social Sciences." *Reviews of Infectious Diseases* 9:980.

Nerenz, David, and Howard Leventhal. 1983. "Self-regulation Theory in Chronic Illness." In Thomas Burish and Laurence Bradley, ed., *Coping with Chronic Illness*. New York: Academic.

Nicholson, William, and Bonita Long. 1990. "Self-esteem, Social Support, Internalized Homophobia, and Coping Strategies of HIV+ Gay Men." *Journal of Consulting and Clinical Psychology* 58 (6):873–876.

Northouse, Laurel. 1984. "The Impact of Cancer on the Family." *International Journal of Psychiatry in Medicine* 14 (3):215.

O'Brien, Mary. 1992. *Living with HIV*. New York: Auburn House.

Organization for Economic Cooperation and Development. 1992. *U.S. Health Care at the Crossroads*. Paris: OECD.

Paringer, Lynn, Kathryn Phillips, and Teh-wei Hu. 1991. "Who Seeks HIV Testing?" *Inquiry* 28:226–35.

Parsons, Talcott. 1951. *The Social System*. Glencoe, Ill.: The Free Press.

Patterson, Bill. 1989. "AIDS in the Workplace." *Training and Development Journal* 43 (2):38–41.

Patton, Cindy. 1985. *Sex and Germs*. Boston: South End.

Patton, Cindy. 1990a. "Why We Can't Get Women and AIDS on the Agenda." *Z Magazine* 3 (12):99–103.

Patton, Cindy. 1990b. *Inventing AIDS*. New York: Routledge.

Patton, Cindy. 1994. *Last Served? Women and the AIDS Pandemic*. London: Taylor and Francis.

Paul, Jay. 1984. "The Bisexual Identity." *Journal of Homosexuality* 9 (2/3):45–63.

Pearlin, Leonard, Shirley Semple and Heather Turner. 1988. "Stress of AIDS Caregiving." *Death Studies* 12:501.

Perkins, Diana, Elizabeth Davidson, Jane Leserman, Duanping Liao, and Dwight Evans. 1993. "Personality Disorder in Patients Infected with HIV." *American Journal of Psychiatry* 150 (2):309–315.

Peterson, John. 1992. "Black Men and Their Same-sex Desires and Behaviors." In Gilbert Herdt, ed., *Gay Culture in America*. Boston: Beacon.

Pierret, Janine. 1992. "Coping With AIDS in Everyday Life." In Michael Pollak, ed., with Geneviève Paicheler and Janine Pierret, *AIDS, A Problem for Sociological Research*. London: Sage.

Plummer, Ken. 1995. *Telling Sexual Stories*. London: Routledge.

Powell-Cope, Gail and Marie Brown. 1992. "Going Public as an AIDS Family Caregiver." *Social Science and Medicine* 34 (5):571–580.

Rabkin, Judith et al. 1990. "Maintenance of Hope in HIV-spectrum Homosexual Men." *American Journal of Psychiatry* 147 (10):1322–1326.

Ragsdale, Diane, Joseph Kotarba, and James Morrow. 1994. "How HIV+ Persons Manage Everyday Life in the Hospital and at Home." *Qualitative Health Research* 4 (4):431–443.

Ritter, Anne. 1989. "AIDS and the Medicinal Power of Work." *Personnel* 66 (11):36–39.

Rowe, William, Gerald Plum, and Clarence Crossman. 1988. "Issues and Problems Confronting the Lovers, Families, and Communities Associated with Persons with AIDS." *Journal of Social Work and Human Sexuality* 6 (2):71.

Sandstrom, Kent. 1990. "Confronting Deadly Disease." *Journal of Contemporary Ethnography* 19 (3):271–294.

Scambler, Graham. 1984. "Perceiving and Coping with Stigmatizing Illness." In Ray Fitzpatrick, John Hinton, Stanton Newman, Graham Scambler, and James Thompson, eds. *The Experience of Illness*. London: Tavistock.

Schellenberg, E. Glenn, Janet Keil, and Sandra Bem. 1995. " 'Innocent Victims' of AIDS." *Journal of Applied Social Psychology* 25(20): 1790–1800.

Schenk, Christopher, and Elaine Bernard. 1992. "Social Unionism." *Social Policy* 23:38–46.

Scheper-Hughes, N. and M. Lock. 1986. "Speaking 'Truth' to Illness." *Medical Anthropology Quarterly* 17 (5):137–139.

Schneider, Beth. 1992. "AIDS and Class, Gender, and Race Relations." In Joan Huber and Beth Schneider, eds. *The Social Context of AIDS*. Newbury Park, CA: Sage.

Schwalbe, Michael, and Clifford Staples. 1992. "Forced Blood Testing." In Joan Huber and Beth Schneider, eds. *The Social Context of AIDS*. Newbury Park, CA: Sage.

Schwartzberg, Steven. 1993. "Struggling for Meaning." *Professional Psychology* 24 (4):483–490.

Sears, Alan. 1991. "AIDS and the Health of Nations." *Critical Sociology* 18 (2) :31–50.

Sedgwick, Eve. 1990. *Epistemology of the Closet.* Berkeley: University of California Press.

Sedgwick, Peter. 1982. *Psycho-Politics.* New York: Harper and Row.

Shelby, R. Dennis. 1992. *If a Partner has AIDS.* New York: Harrington Park Press.

Siegel, Karolynn, and Beatrice Krauss. 1991. "Living with HIV Infection." *Journal of Health and Social Behavior* 32 (1):17–32.

Siegel, Karolynn, Victoria Raveis and Daniel Karus. 1994. "Psychological Well-Being of Gay Men with AIDS." *Social Science and Medicine* 39 (11):1555–1563.

Singer, Merrill. 1994. "AIDS and the Health Crisis of the U.S. Urban Poor." *Social Science and Medicine* 39 (7):931–948.

Smith, George. 1994. "Palliative Care in Toronto for People with AIDS." *Journal of Palliative Care* 10 (2):46–50.

Solomon, George, and Lydia Temoshok. 1987. "A Psychoneuroimmunologic Perspective on AIDS Research." *Journal of Applied Social Psychology* 17 (1):286.

Sontag, Susan. 1978. *Illness as Metaphor.* New York: Farrar, Strauss and Giroux.

Spillman, Brenda. 1992. "The Impact of Being Uninsured on the Utilization of Basic Health Care Services." *Inquiry* 29:457–466.

Strauss, Anselm. 1975. *Chronic Illness and the Quality of Life.* St Louis: Mosby.

Stulberg, Ian, and Stephan Buckingham. 1988. "Parallel Issues for AIDS Patients, Families, and Others." *Social Casework* 69 (6):355–359.

Taussig, Michael T. 1992. "Reification and the Consciousness of the Patient." *Social Science and Medicine* 14B:3–13.

Tedlow, Richard, and Michele Marram. 1991. "A Case of AIDS." *Harvard Business Review* 69 (6):14–25.

Tesh, Sylvia. 1988. *Hidden Arguments.* New Brunswick, NJ: Rutgers University Press.

Thompson, Edward P. 1968. *The Making of the English Working Class.* Harmondsworth: Penguin.

Tiblier, Kay. 1987. "Intervening with Families of Young Adults with AIDS." In Maureen Leahey and Lorraine Wright, eds. *Families and Life-Threatening Illness.* Springhouse, PA: Springhouse Corporation.

Trice, Ashton. 1988. "Posttraumatic Stress Syndrome-like Symptoms Among AIDS Caregivers." *Psychological Reports* 63:656.

Triplet, Rodney, and David Sugarman. 1987. "Reactions to AIDS Victims." *Personality and Social Psychology Bulletin* 13:265–274.

Viney, Linda, and Lynne Bousfield. 1991. "Narrative Analysis." *Social Science and Medicine* 32 (7):757–765.

Vogel, Lise. 1990. "Debating Difference." *Feminist Studies* 16 (1).

Watney, Simon. 1987. *Policing Desire.* London: Comedia.

Weisman, Avery. 1979. *Coping With Cancer.* New York: McGraw-Hill.

Weisman, Avery, and J. William Worden. 1976–77. "The Existential Plight in Cancer." *International Journal of Psychiatry in Medicine* 7 (1):1.

Weitz,, Rose. 1987. "The Interview As Legacy." *Hastings Center Report* 17 (3):21–23.

Weitz, Rose. 1989. "Uncertainty and the Lives of Persons with AIDS." *Journal of Health and Social Behavior* 30 (Sept):270.

Weitz, Rose. 1990. "Living with the Stigma of AIDS." *Qualitative Sociology* 13 (1):23–38.

Weitz, Rose. 1991. *Life With AIDS.* New Brunswick, NJ: Rutgers University Press.

Weston, Kath. 1991. *Families We Choose.* New York: Columbia University Press.

Williams, R. Jane, and William Stafford. 1991. "Silent Casualties." *Journal of Counselling and Development* 69 (5):423–427.

Williams, Walter. 1986. *The Spirit and the Flesh.* Boston: Beacon.

Wolcott, Deane et al. 1986. "Illness Concerns, Attitudes Towards Homosexuality, and Social Support in Gay Men with AIDS." *General Hospital Psychiatry* 8:395.

Wolf, Thomas, et al. 1991. "Relationship of Coping Style to Affective State and Perceived Social Support in Asymptomatic and Symptomatic HIV-infected Persons." *Journal of Clinical Psychiatry* 52 (4):171–174.

Wortman, Camille, and Christine Dunkel-Schetter. 1979. "Interpersonal Relationships and Cancer." *Journal of Social Issues* 35 (1):120.

Wright, Jerome. 1993. "African-American Male Sexual Behavior and the Risk for HIV Infection." *Human Organization* 52 (4):421–431.

Yelin, Edward, Ruth Greenblatt, Harry Hollander, and Joan McMaster. 1991. "The Impact of HIV-Related Illness on Employment." *American Journal of Public Health* 81 (1):79–84.

INDEX